PENGUIN BOOKS

THE DESPERATE WOMAN'S GUIDE TO DIET AND EXERCISE

GW00363586

A mid-century product of Tyneside, Jo Nesbitt went to a convent school, then London University, where the college shrink interpreted the giant nuns which frequented her dreams as 'phallic symbols', an insight which she has always treasured. Freelance since 1978, her work has appeared in *Time Out*, the *New Statesman*, *Spare Rib*, Open University and many educational publications. After moving to Holland in 1981, she published a number of books, of which *The Modern Ladies' Compendium* (cartoons) and *The Great Escape of Doreen Potts* (for children) also appeared in English. *The Desperate Woman's Guide to Therapy* (with Gillian Reeve) is also available in Penguin.

The Desperate Woman's Guide to Diet and Exercise

Jo Nesbitt

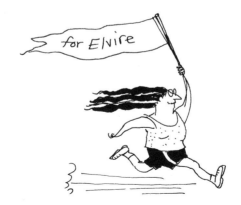

PENGUIN BOOKS

PENGUIN BOOKS

Published by the Penguin Group
Penguin Books Ltd, 27 Wrights Lane, London W8 5TZ, England
Penguin Putnam Inc., 375 Hudson Street, New York, New York 10014, USA
Penguin Books Australia Ltd, Ringwood, Victoria, Australia
Penguin Books Canada Ltd, 10 Alcorn Avenue, Toronto, Ontario, Canada M4V 3B2
Penguin Books (NZ) Ltd, Private Bag, 102902, NSMC, Auckland, New Zealand

Penguin Books Ltd, Registered Offices: Harmondsworth, Middlesex, England

Published by Penguin Books 1998
10 9 8 7 6 5 4 3 2 1

Set in Monotype Photina
Printed in England by Clays Ltd, St Ives plc

Contents

Good Resolutions

I've decided to cut down on your rations

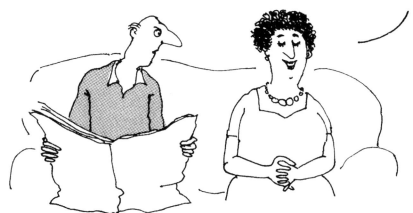

so how come
you lost so much
weight ?

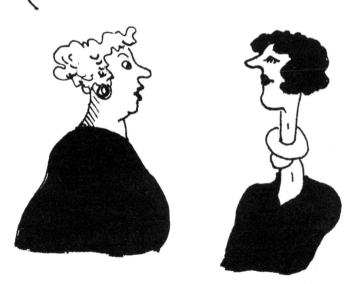

let's see...
if I cut down to
1000 calories a day...
work out at the gym,
swim twice a week,
do yoga...
I should reach
my ideal
weight by...
...April
2007...

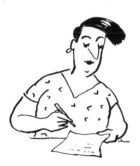

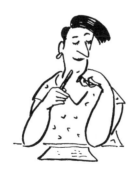

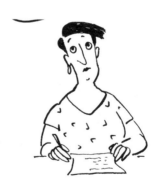

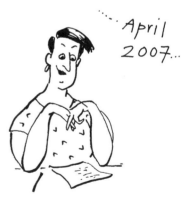

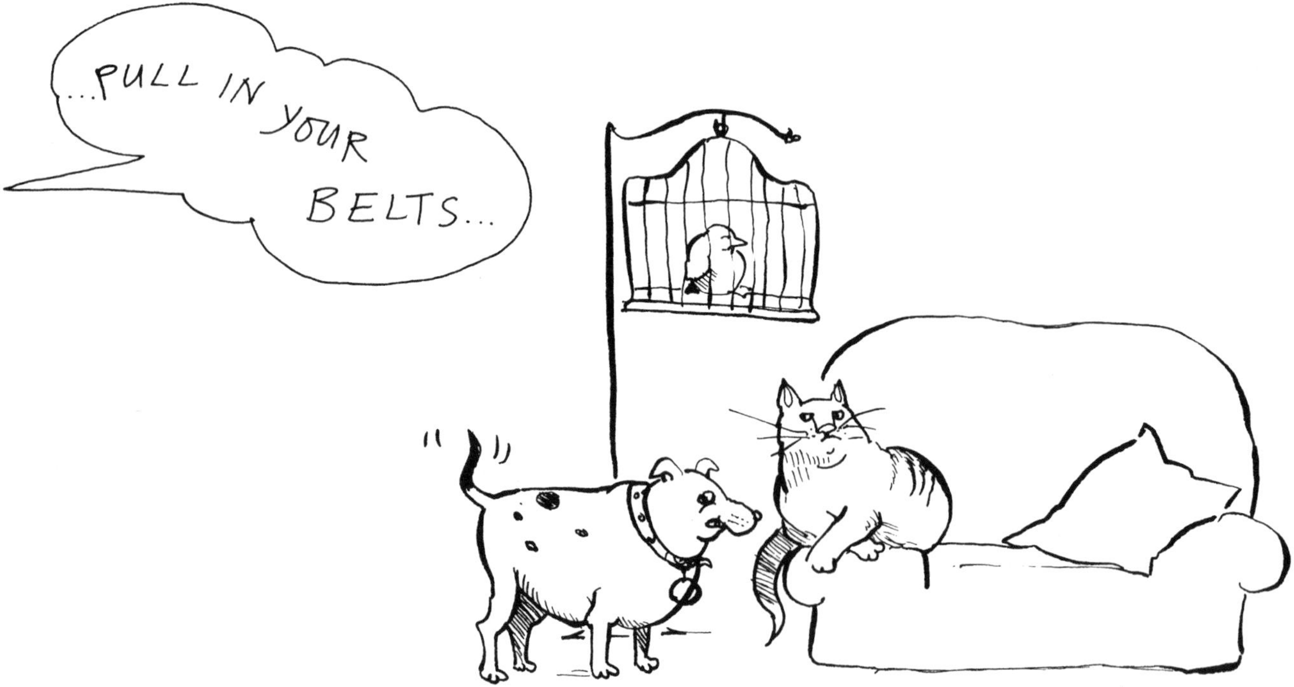
...PULL IN YOUR BELTS...

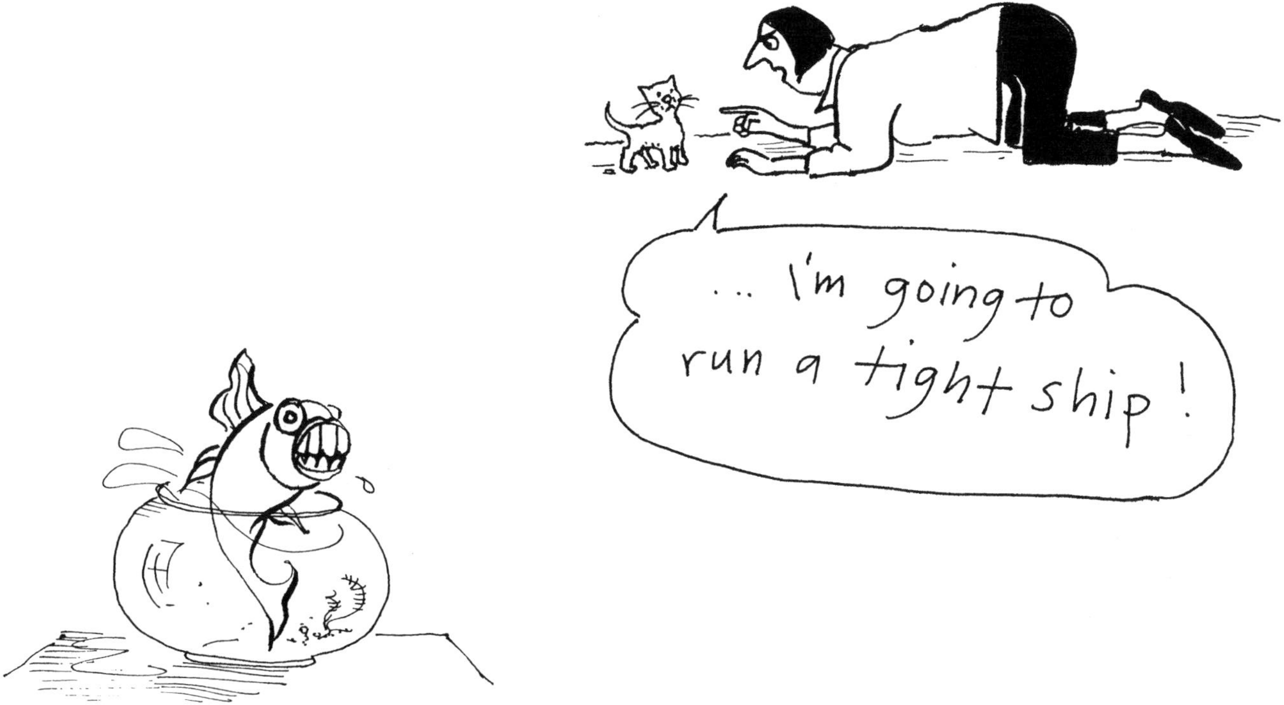
... I'm going to run a tight ship!

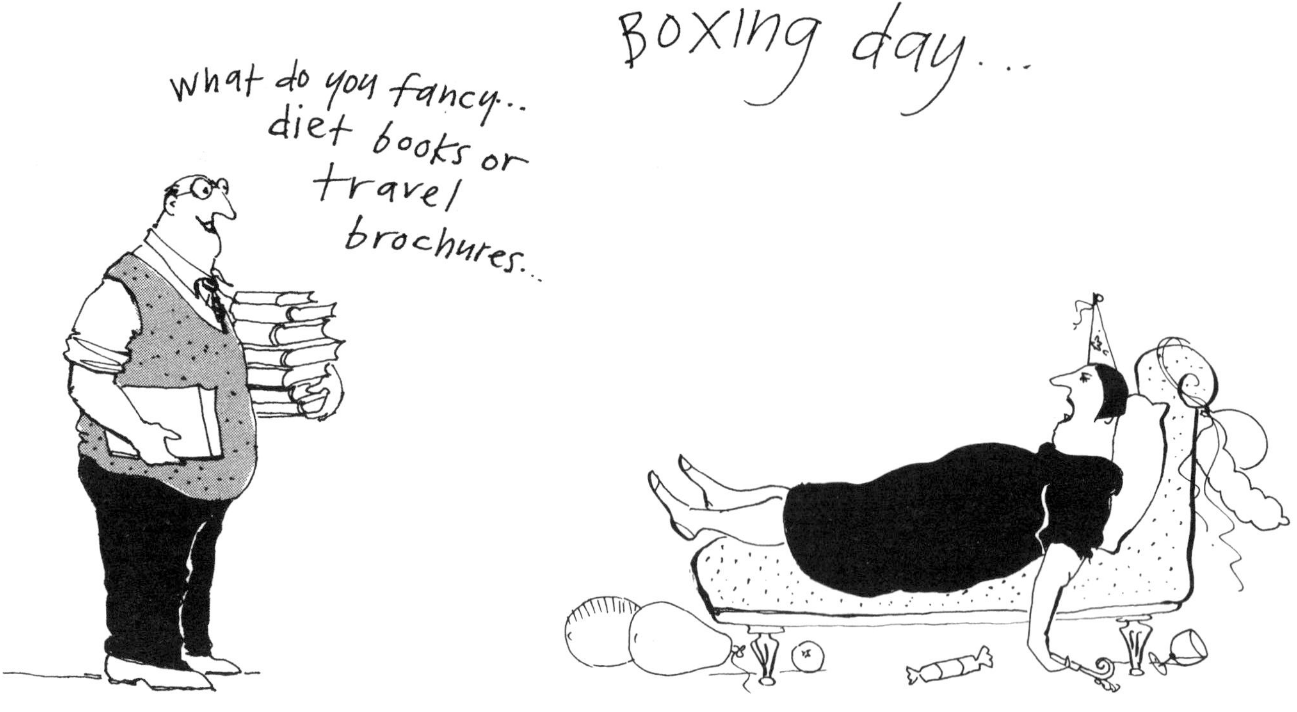
Boxing day...
what do you fancy... diet books or travel brochures...

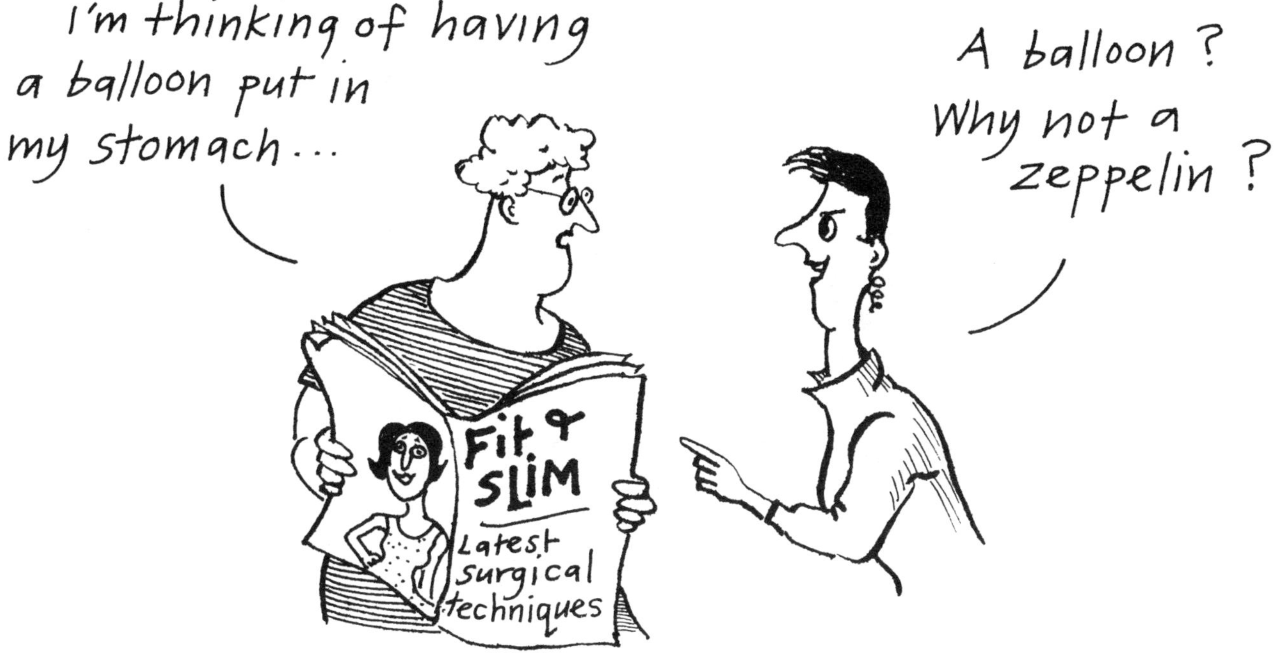
I'm thinking of having a balloon put in my stomach...
A balloon? Why not a zeppelin?
Fit & SLIM
Latest surgical techniques

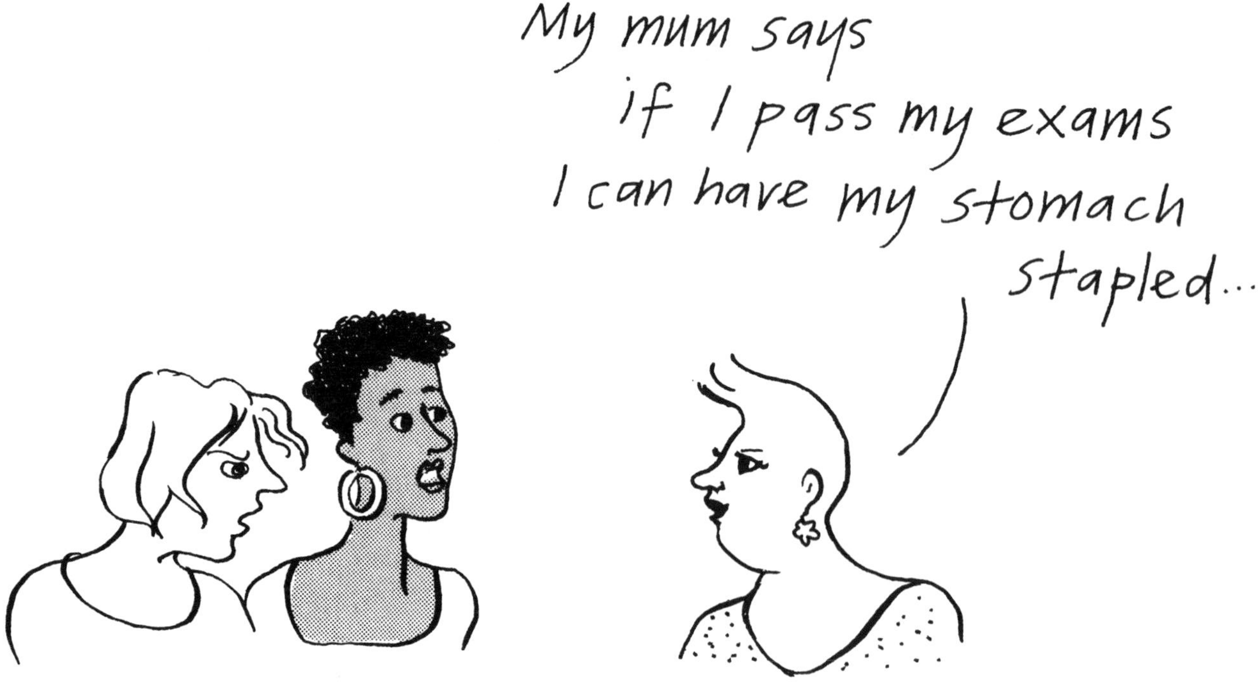
My mum says if I pass my exams I can have my stomach stapled...

Excuses, excuses

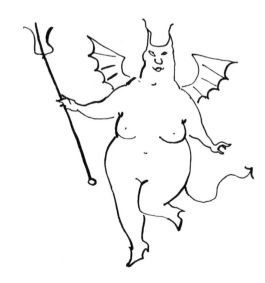

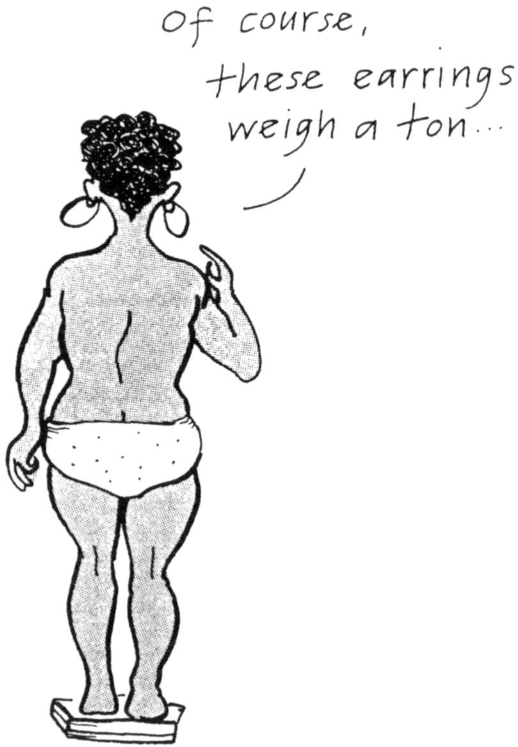
Of course,
these earrings
weigh a ton...

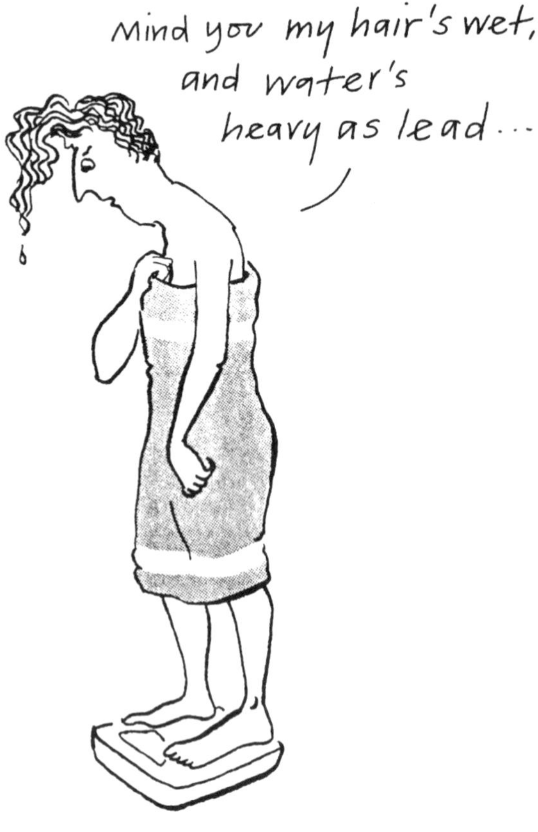
Mind you my hair's wet,
and water's
heavy as lead...

...Heavy bones...?

I'd like one like this, but in a heavier bone size...

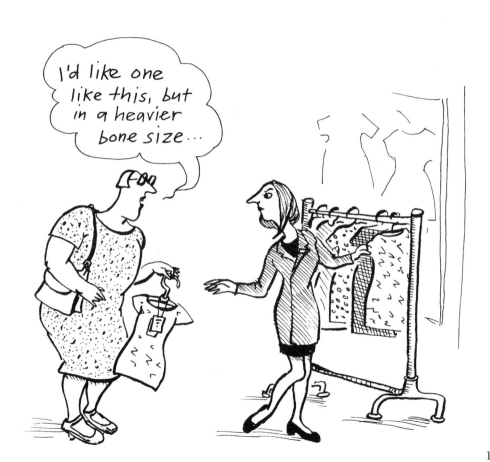

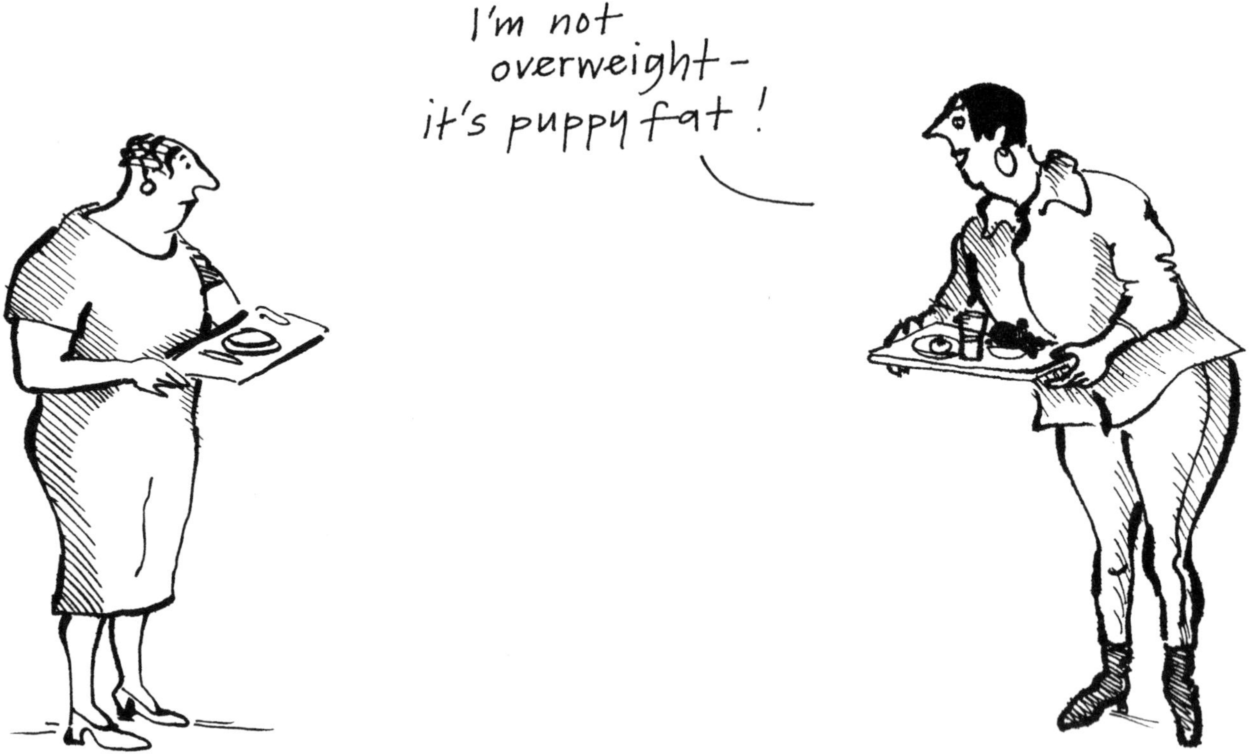
I'm not overweight - it's puppy fat!

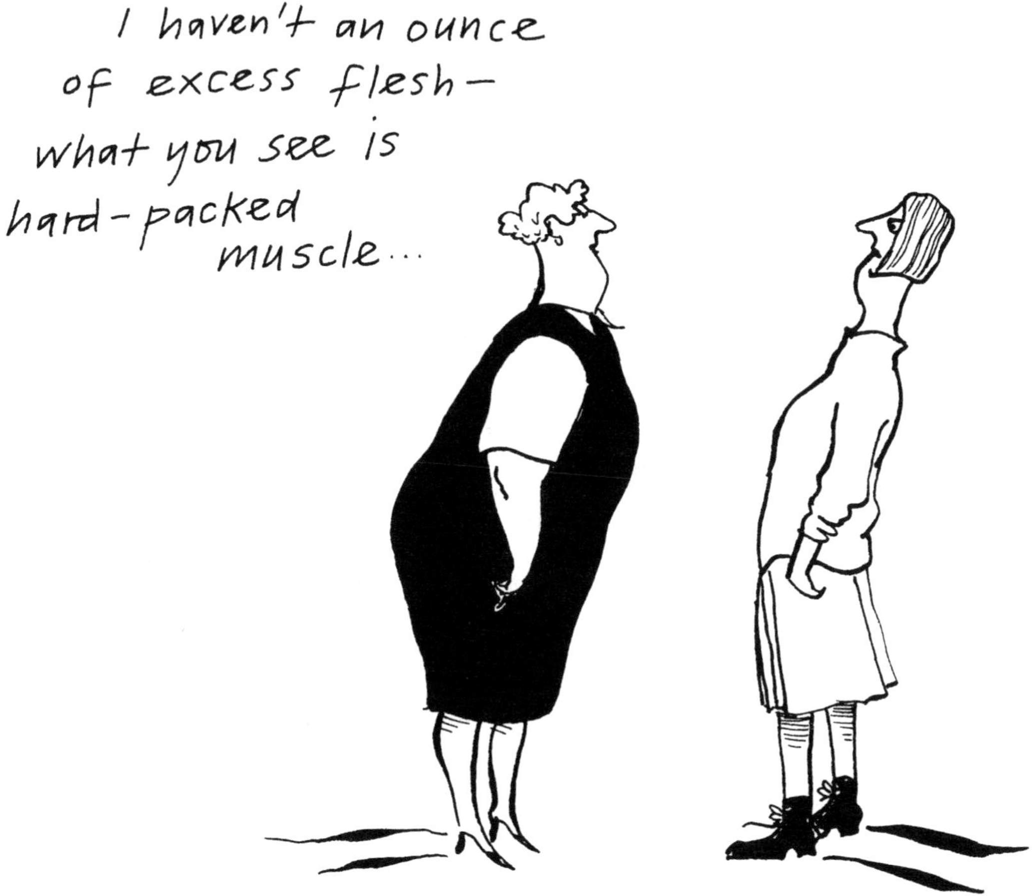
I haven't an ounce of excess flesh– what you see is hard-packed muscle...

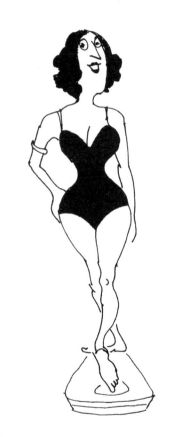
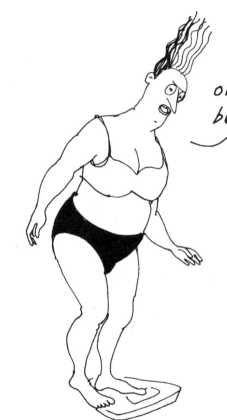

I always put on
one and a half stone
before a period...

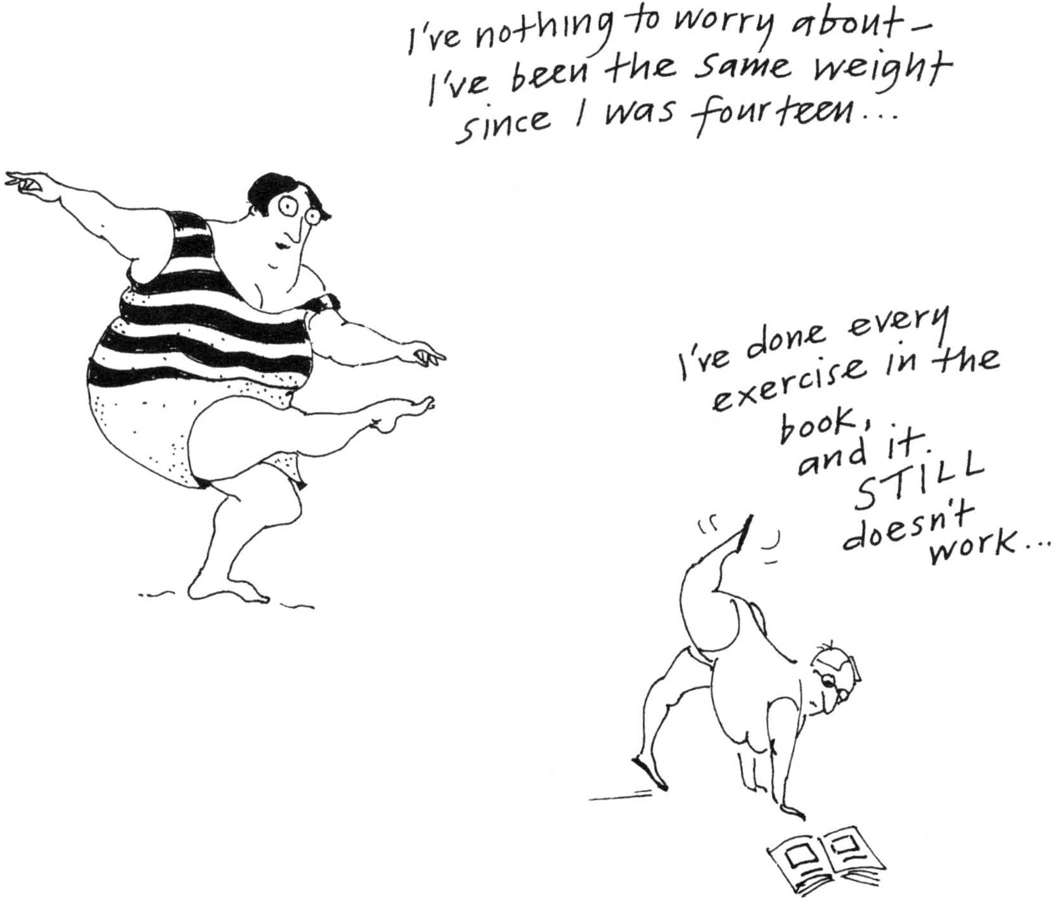
I've nothing to worry about – I've been the same weight since I was fourteen...
I've done every exercise in the book, and it STILL doesn't work...

It's not so fattening if you eat it standing up !

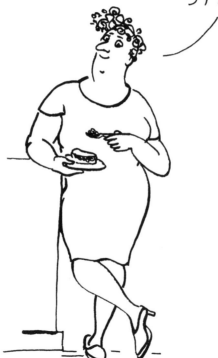

fat legs run in our family...

it's as simple as that!

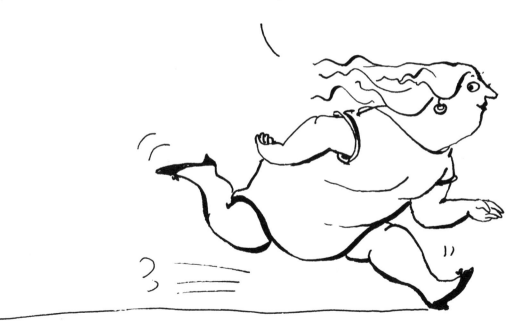

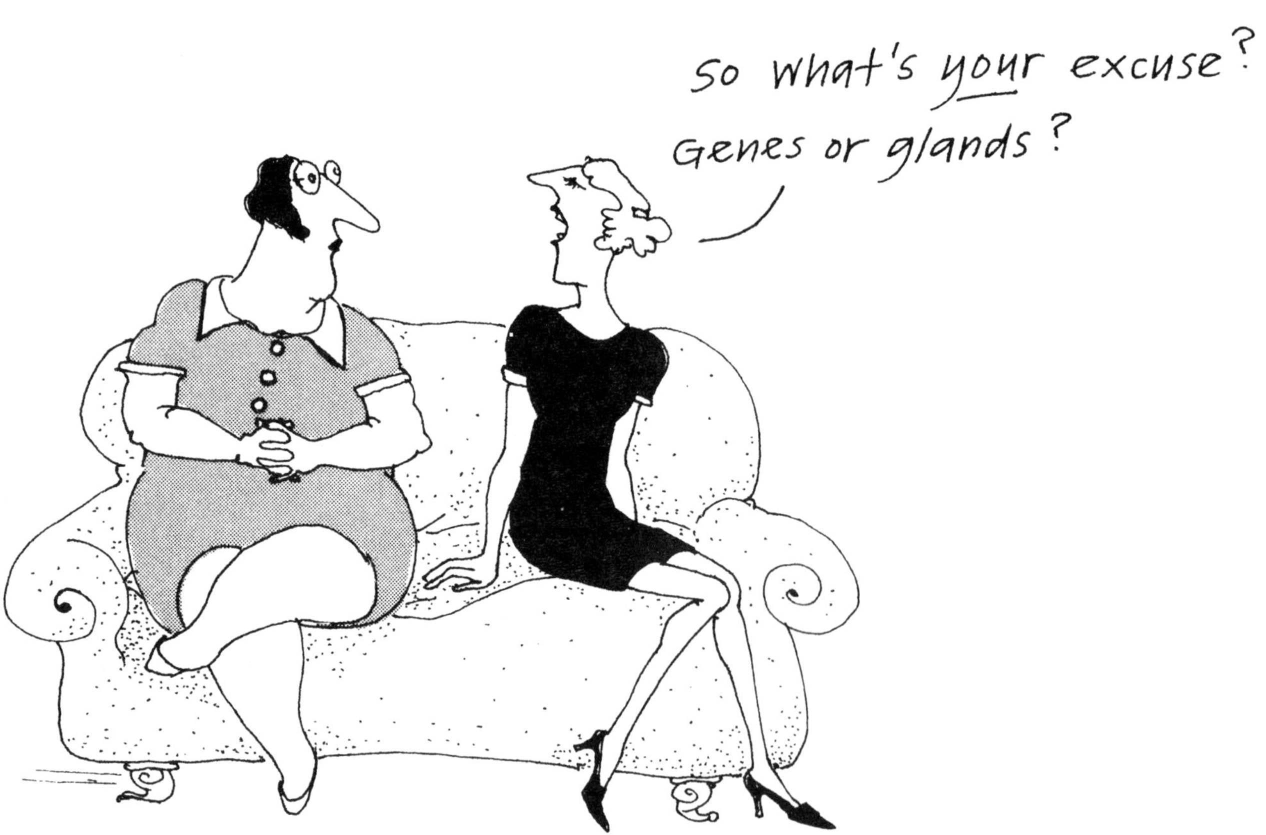
So what's your excuse?
Genes or glands?

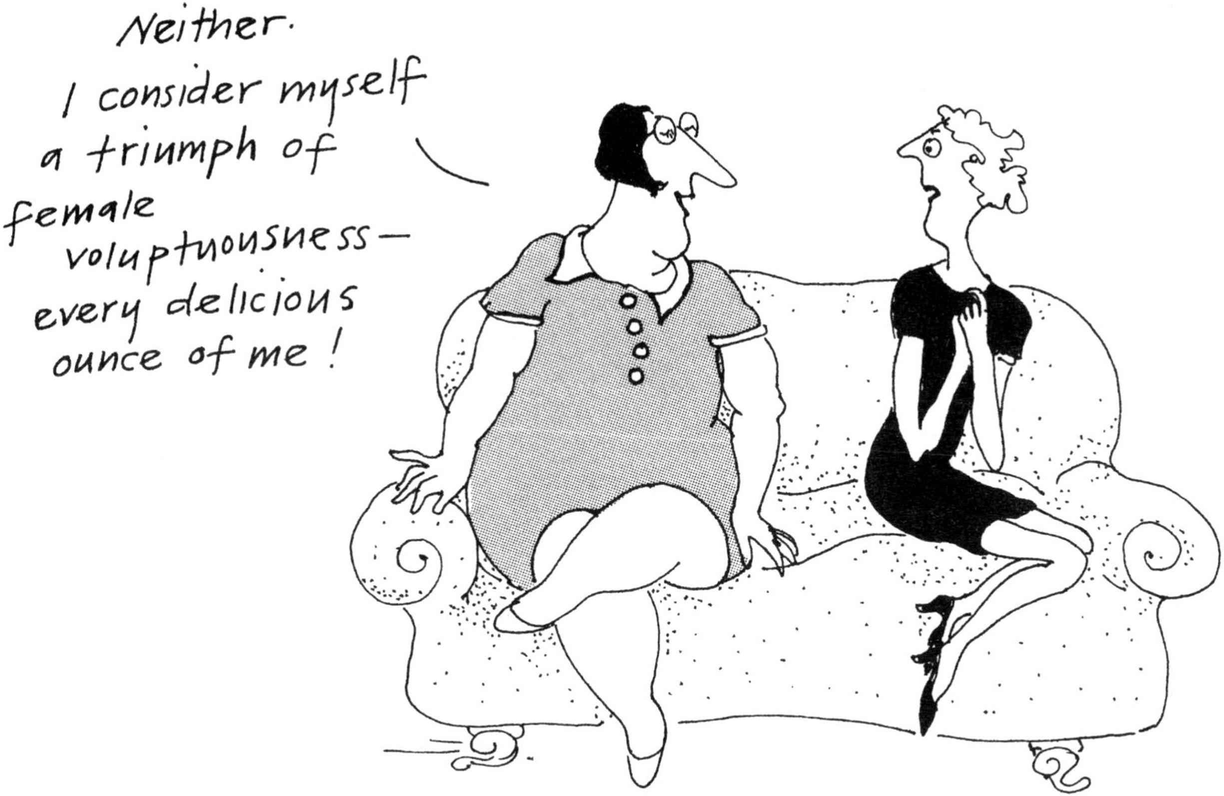
Neither. I consider myself a triumph of female voluptuousness— every delicious ounce of me!

It's not BLUBBER, it's a SAFETY PRECAUTION... Keep me afloat for hours in Arctic waters, this would....

I'm laying down fat reserves for lean times ahead
I think of it as an investment

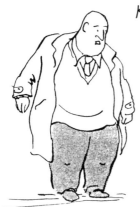

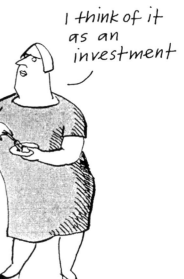

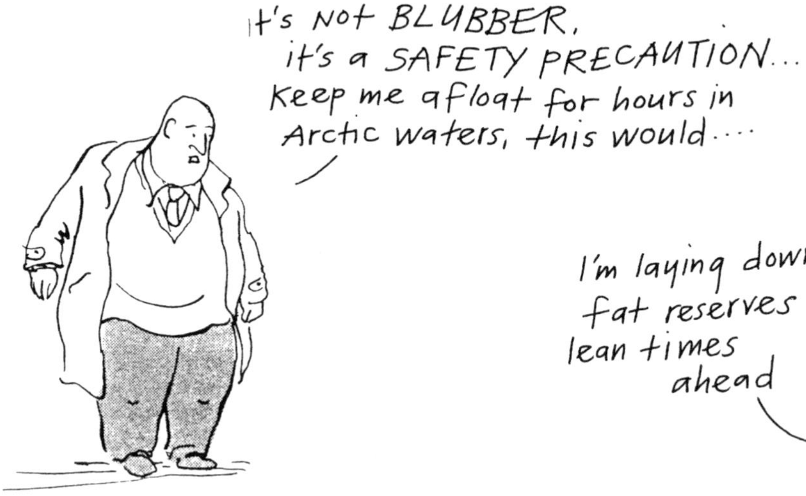

Diet

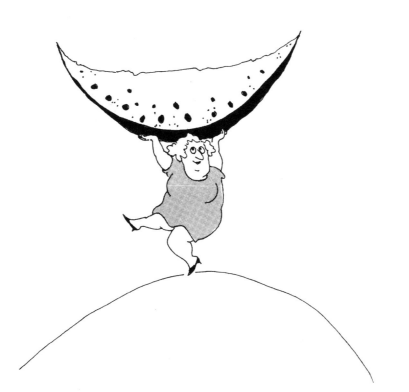

...Here you are - a healthy nine-pound girl...
Nine pounds?

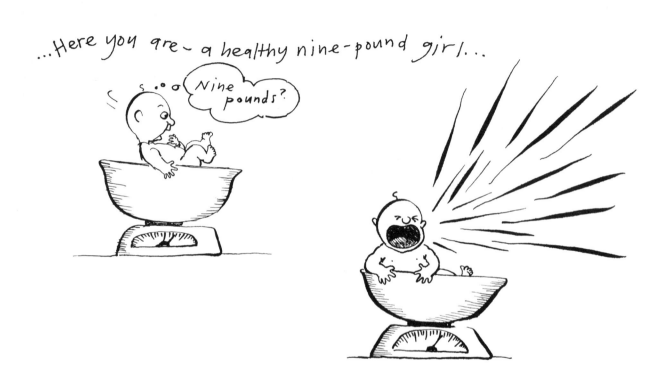

Birth of a Future Dieter

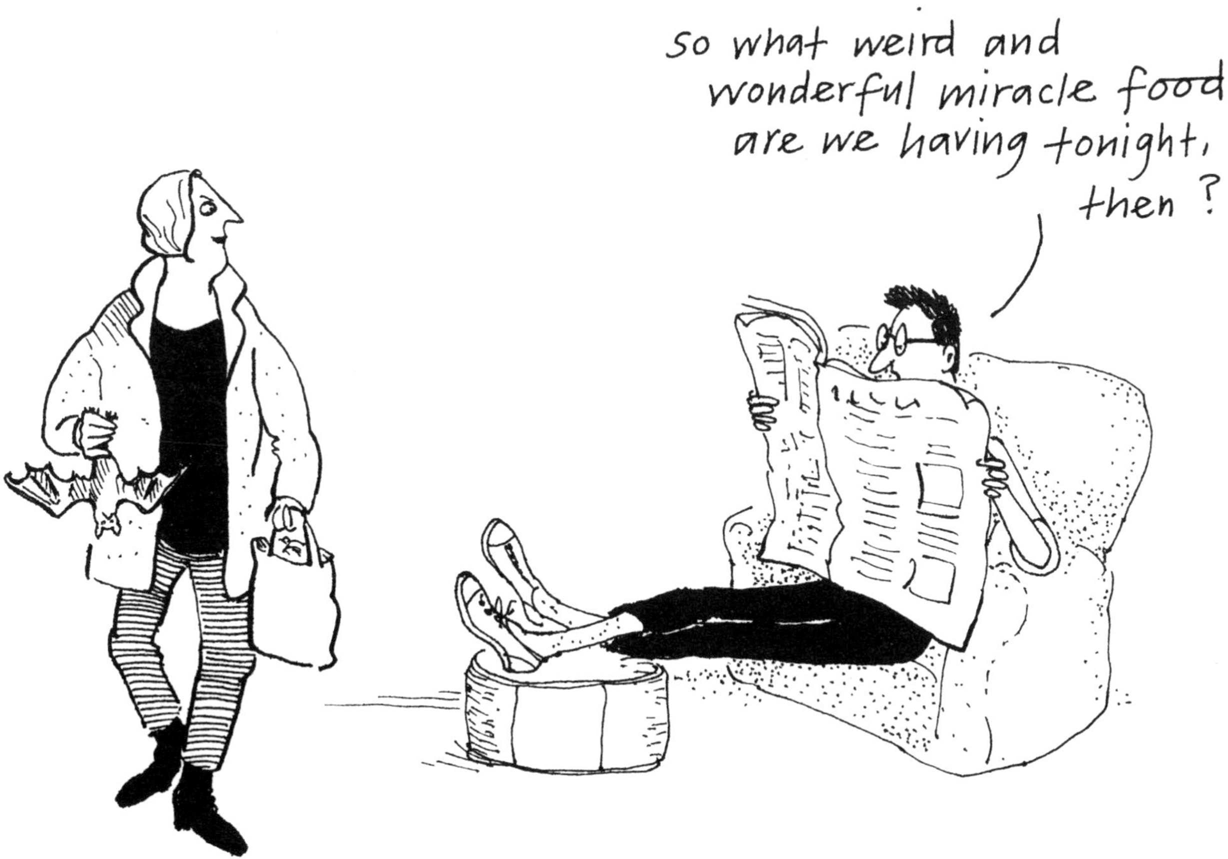
so what weird and wonderful miracle food are we having tonight, then ?

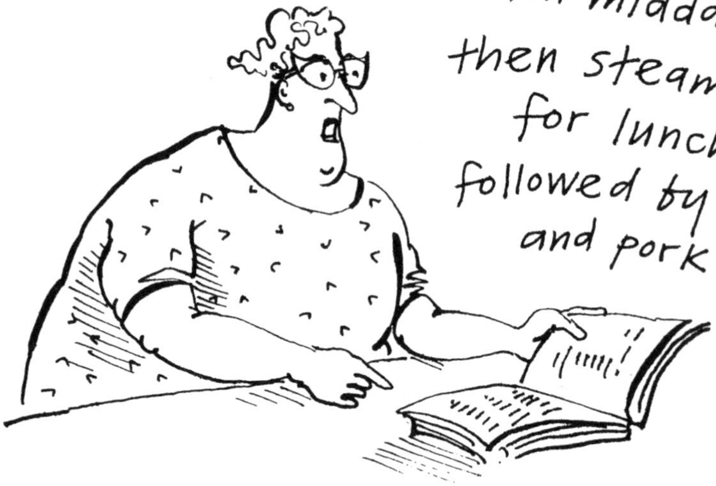

It's quite simple, really:
you have nothing but fruit
till midday,
then steamed vegetables
for lunch,
followed by a pound of lard
and pork scratchings for
dinner...

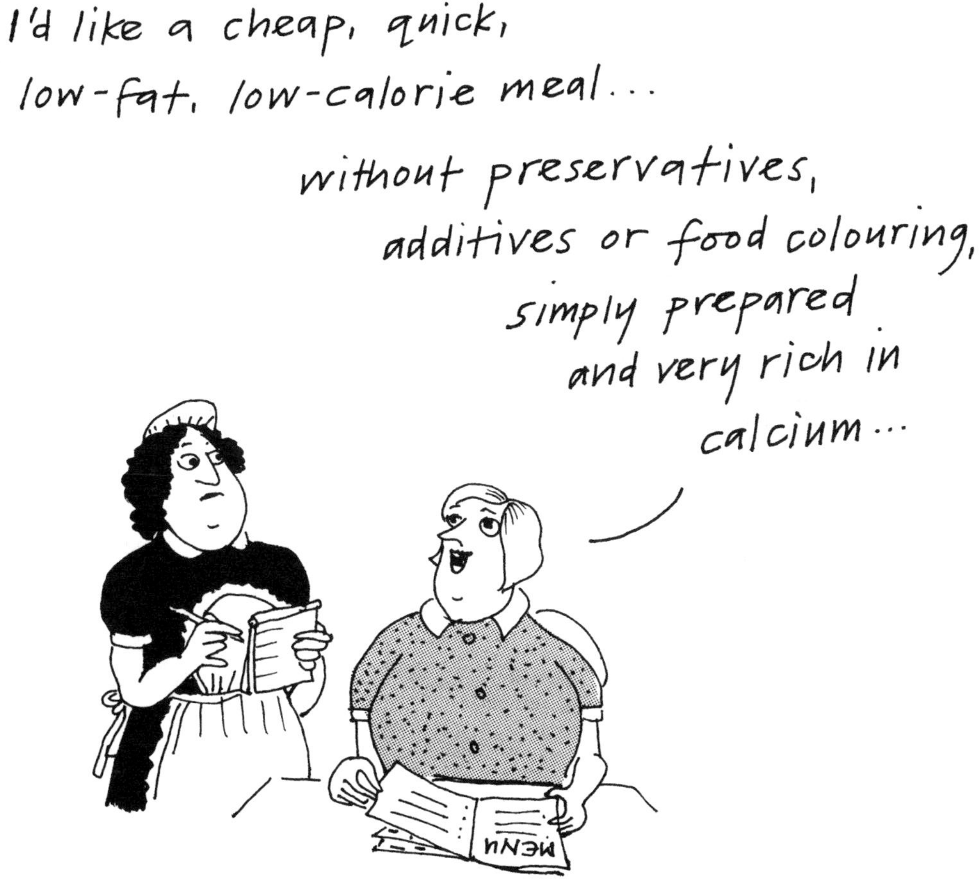
I'd like a cheap, quick, low-fat, low-calorie meal...
without preservatives, additives or food colouring, simply prepared and very rich in calcium...

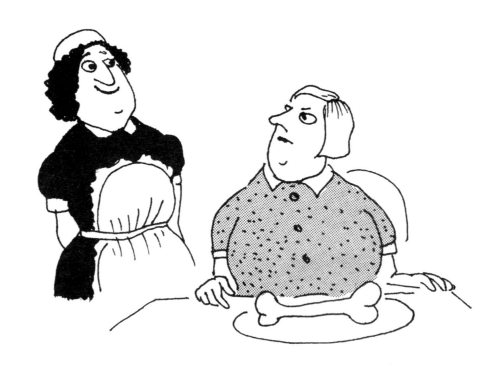

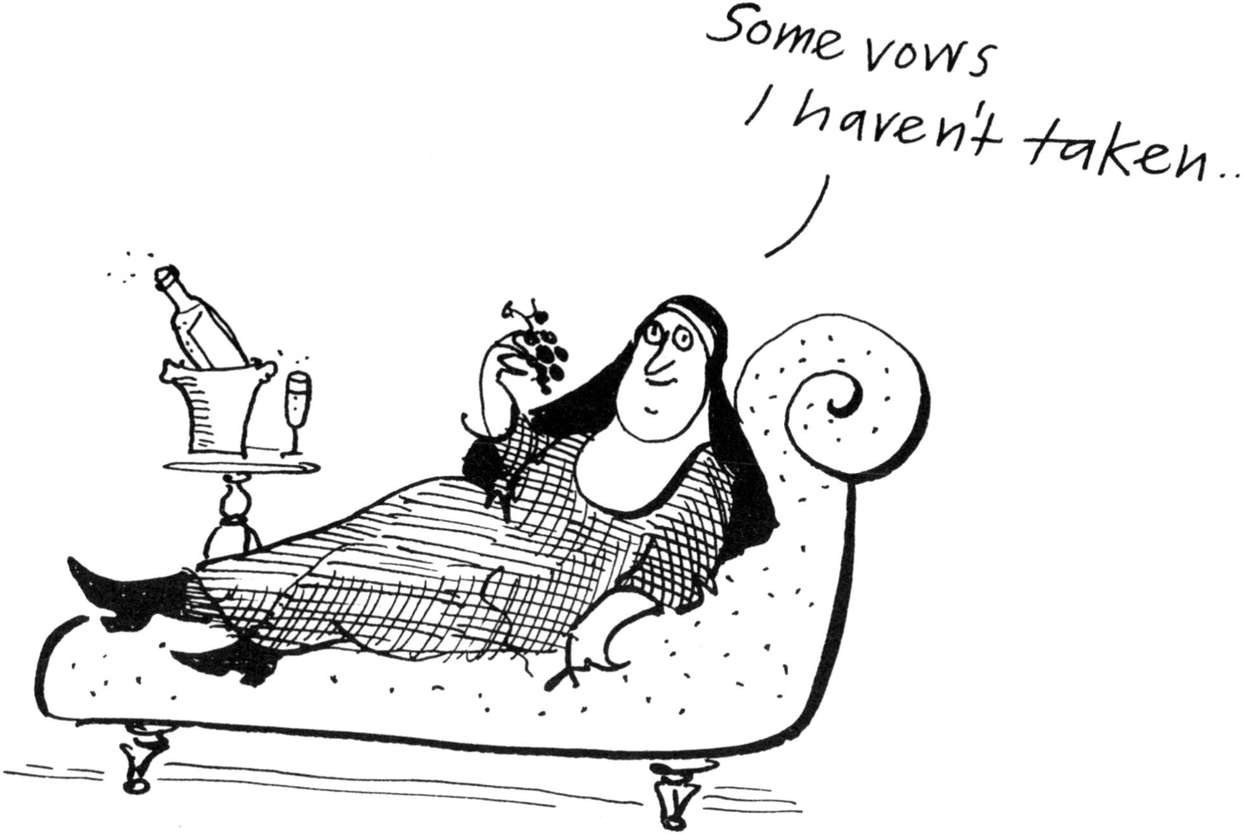
Some vows
I haven't taken...

NEW! with added FOOD!

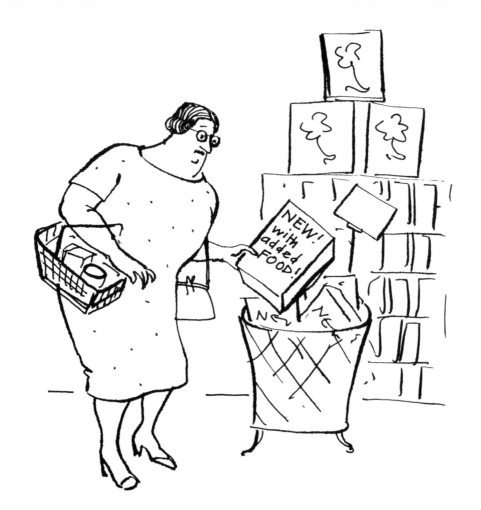

I've put on simply POUNDS over Christmas...

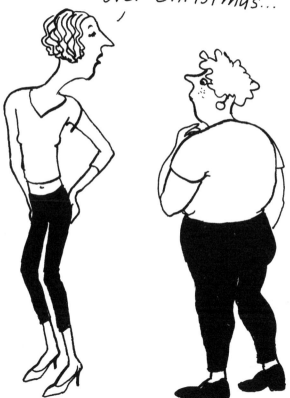

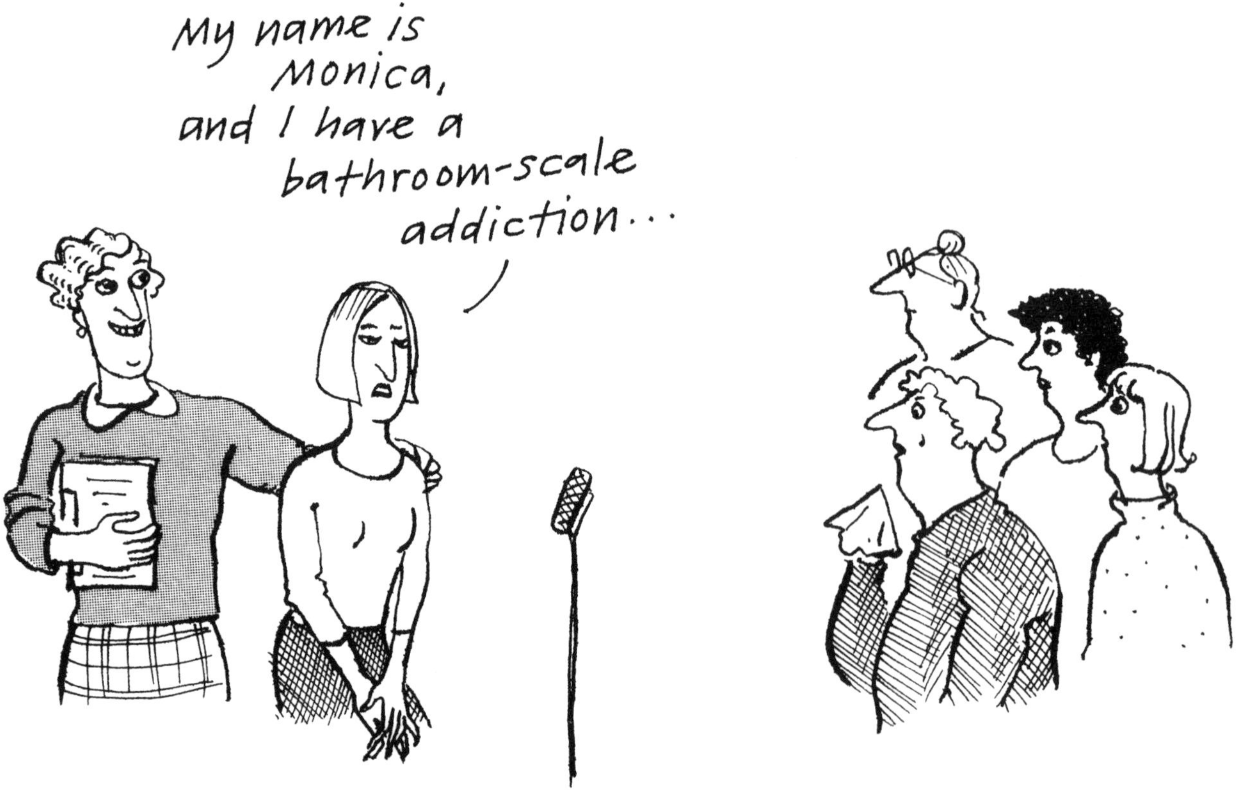
My name is Monica, and I have a bathroom-scale addiction...

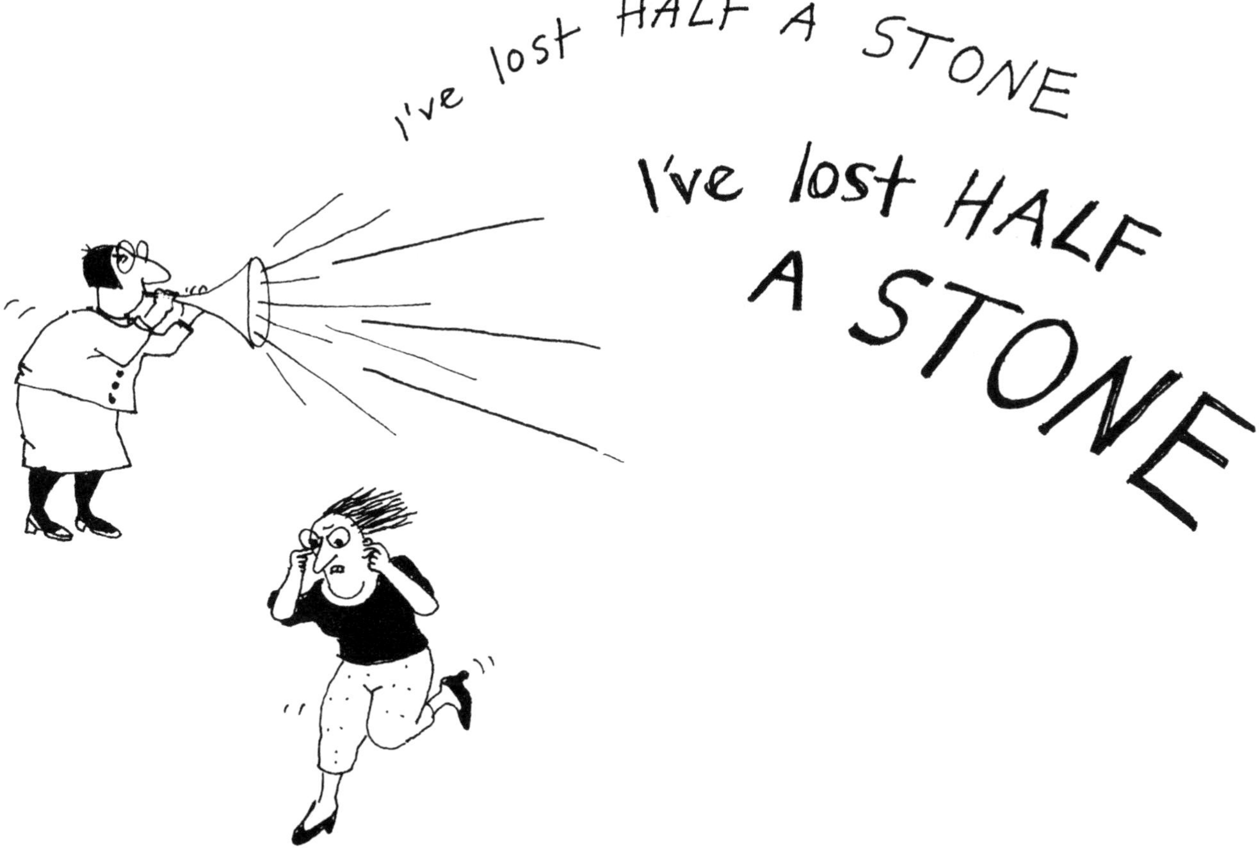
I've lost HALF A STONE
I've lost HALF A STONE

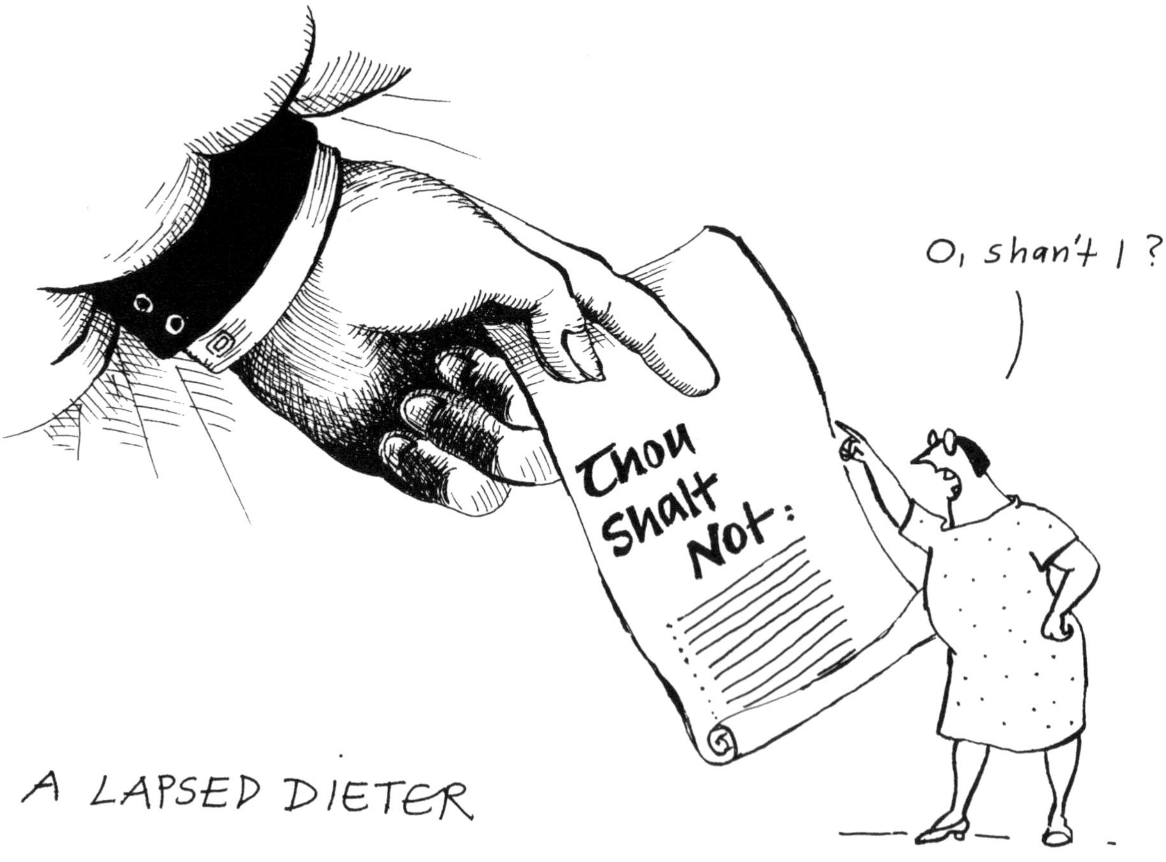
Thou Shalt Not:
O, shan't I ?

A LAPSED DIETER

I'm doing GCSE's
in Dieting,
Aerobics and
    Applied Make-Up...

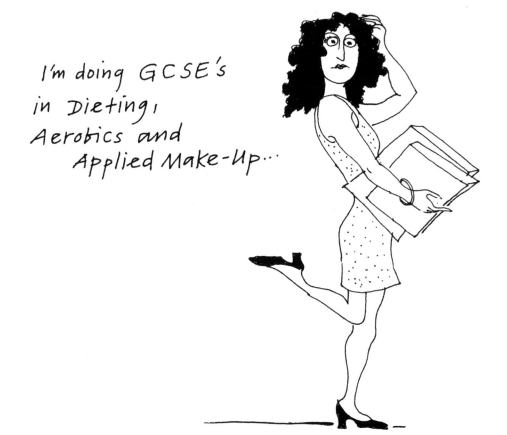

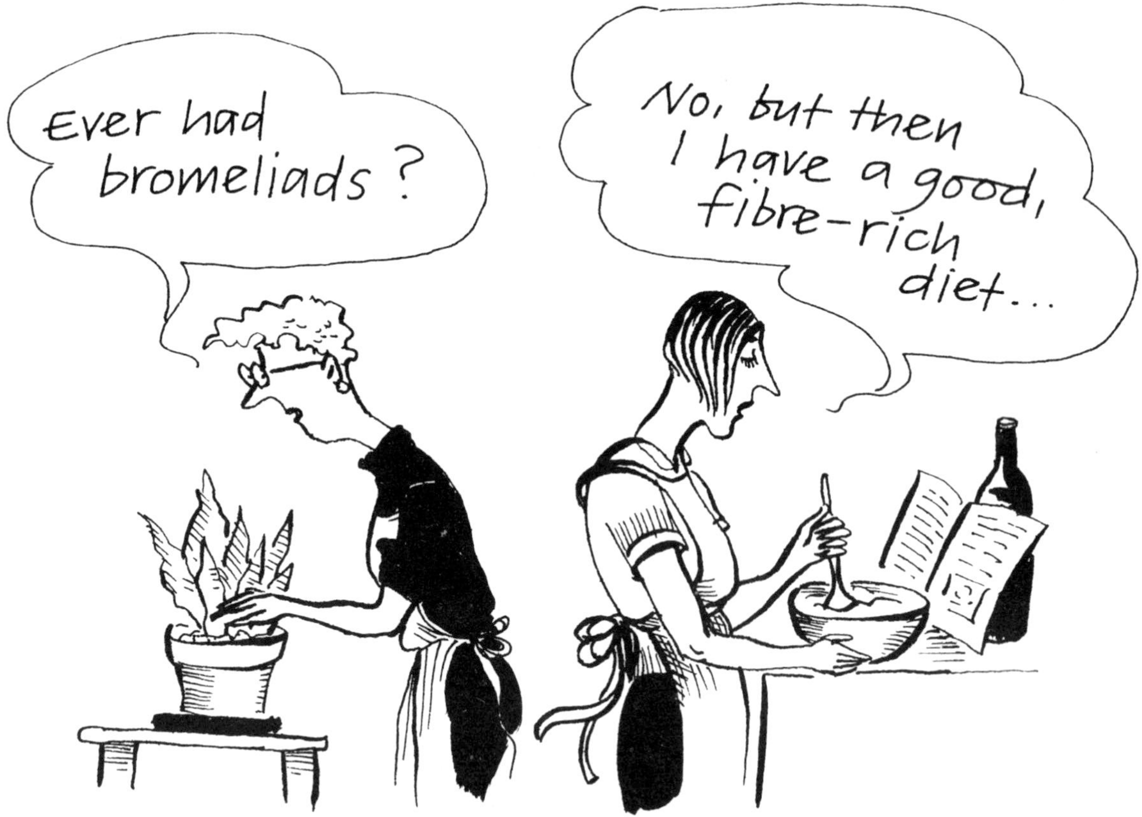
Ever had bromeliads ?
No, but then I have a good, fibre-rich diet...

I tell you, George, I will not put POISON into my system...
I say, Daphne old girl, aren't you going it a bit strong?

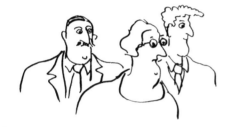

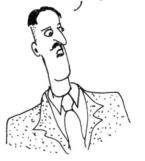

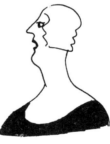

The Woman Who Refused To Combine Protein and Carbohydrate at the same meal...

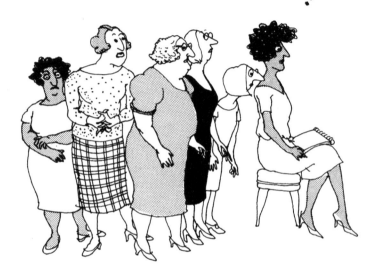
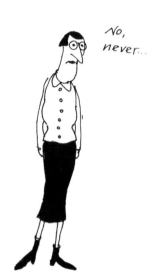

The Woman Who Had Never Been on a Diet...

36

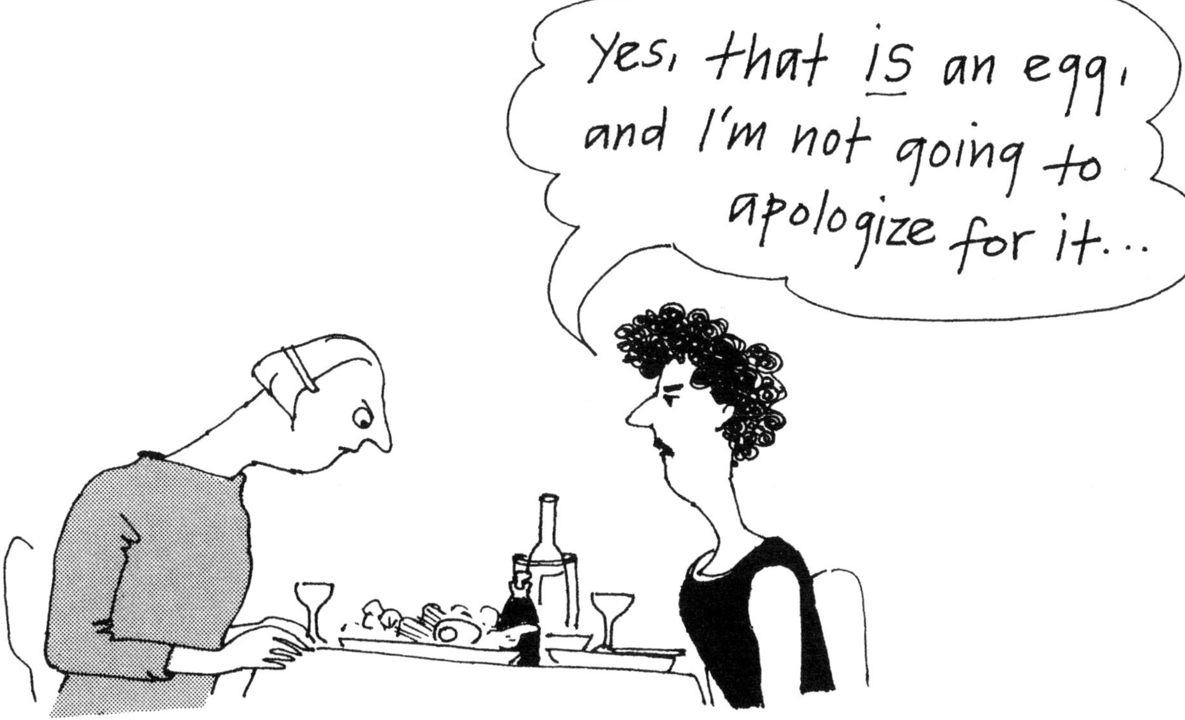
Yes, that IS an egg, and I'm not going to apologize for it...

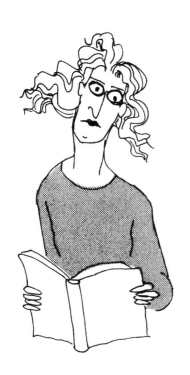

← A woman who is NOT thinking about chocolate...

NOW - which one has
the least
cholesterol ?

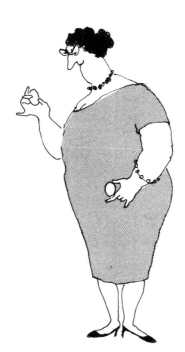

I drink pure lemon juice before every meal to re-educate my taste-buds....
Mine have learning difficulties!

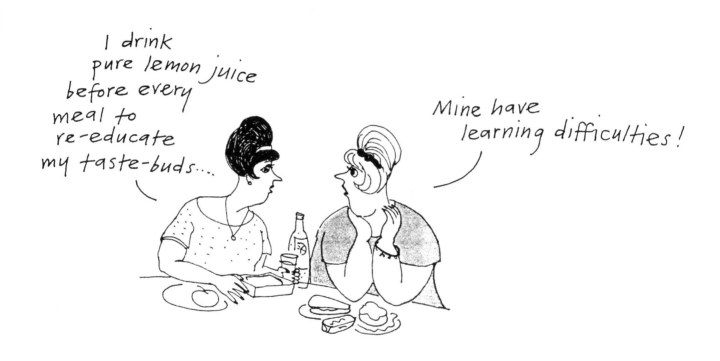

Dieting 1960s style

Exercise

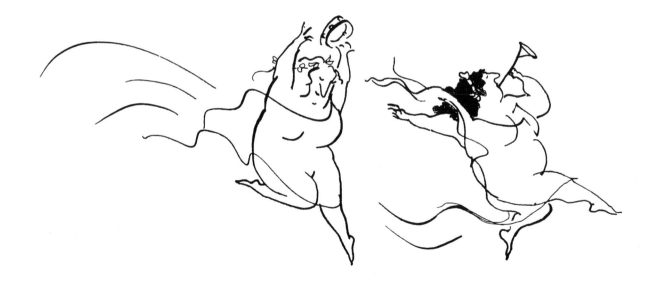

Don't forget ...

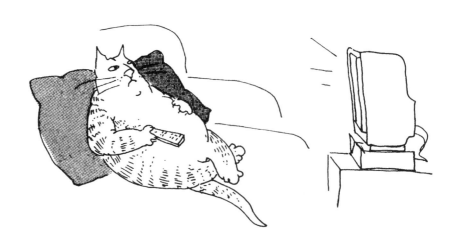

... the whole family will want to join in your new, healthier regime....

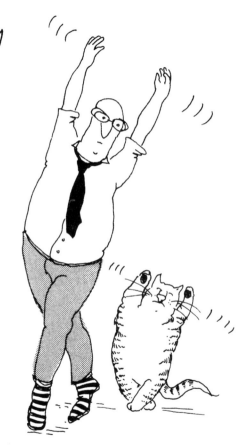

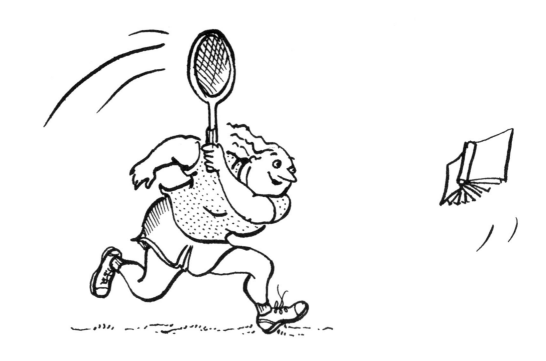

making the Best use of your Diet Book

CHOCS

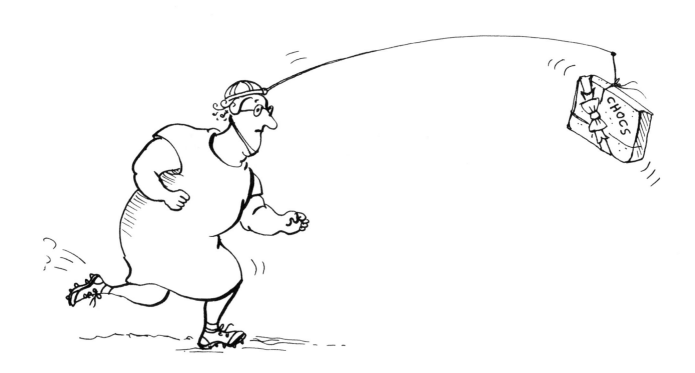

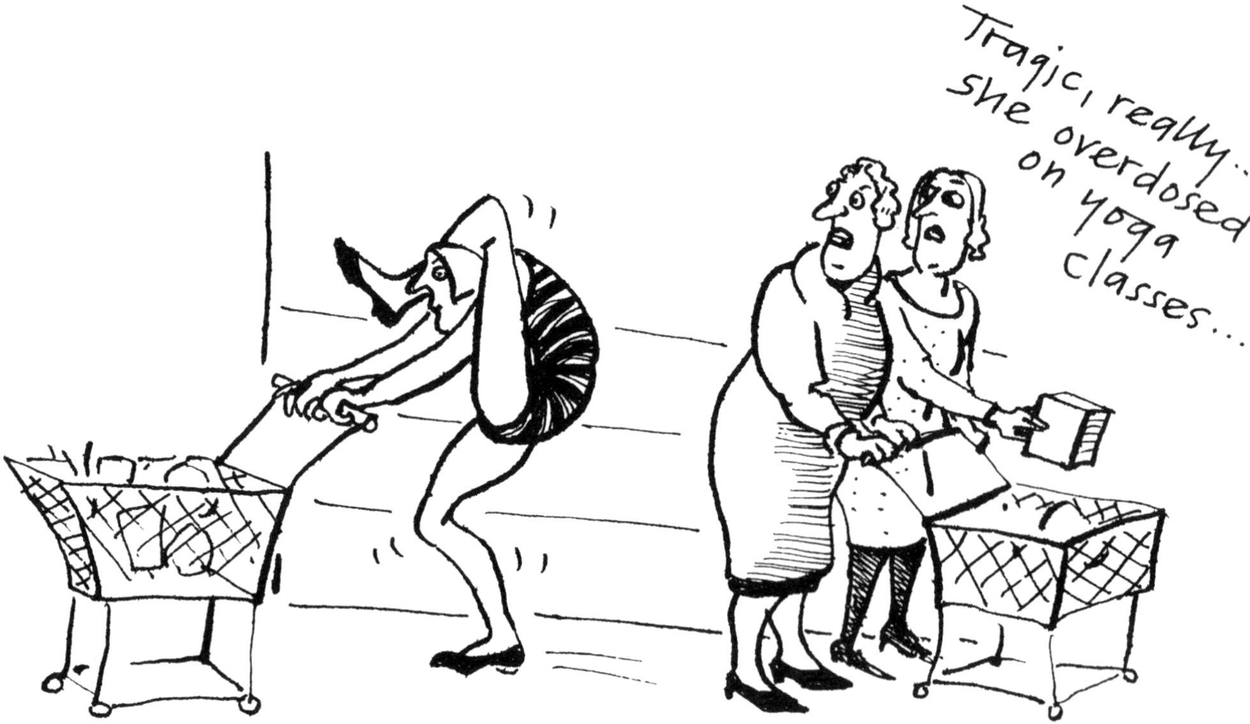
Tragic, really...
she overdosed
on yoga
classes...

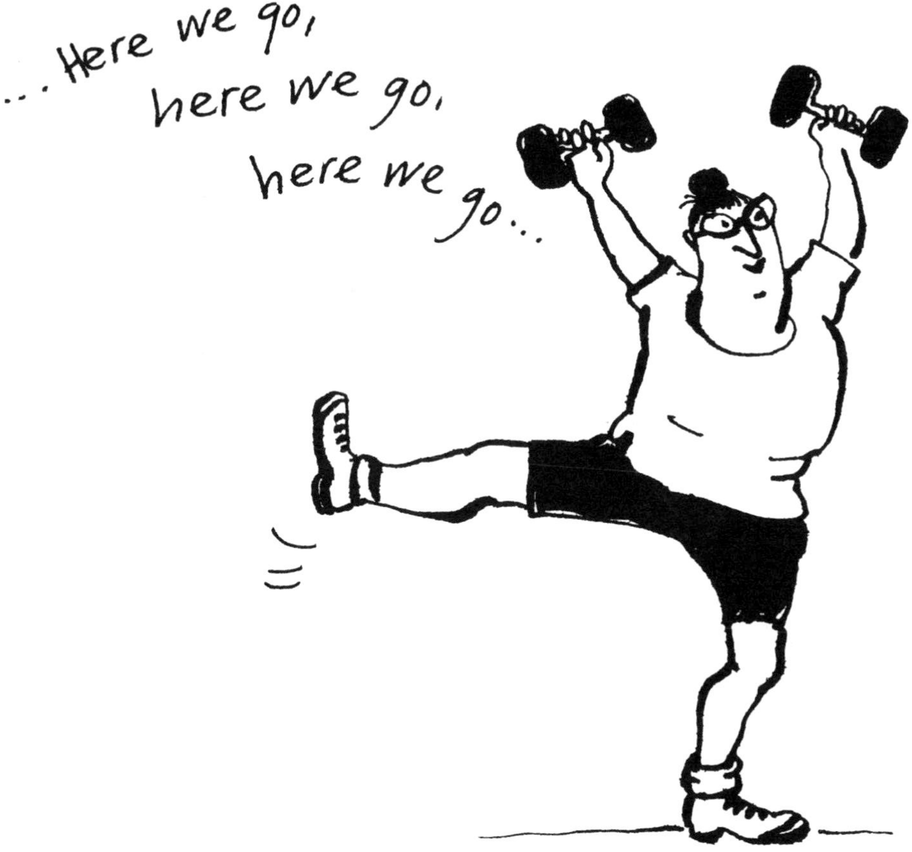
...Here we go,
here we go,
here we go...

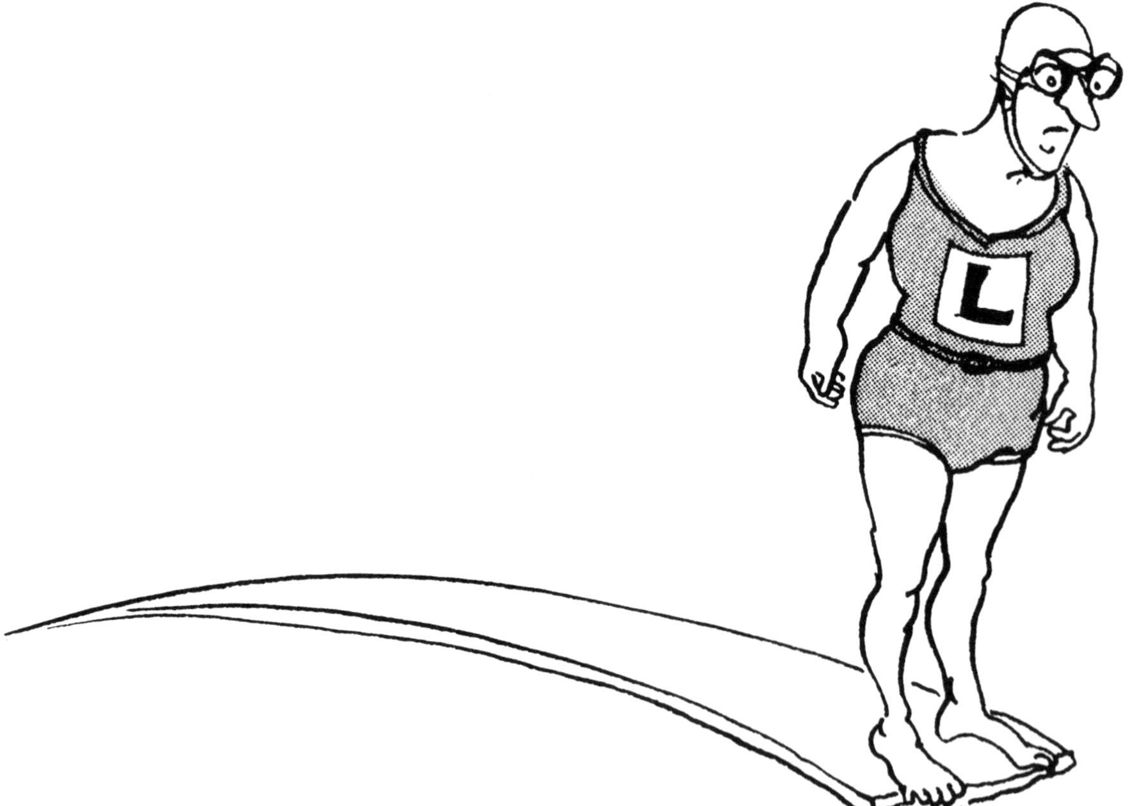
L

friends will admire
the new balanced you...

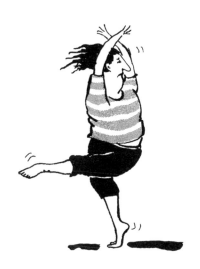

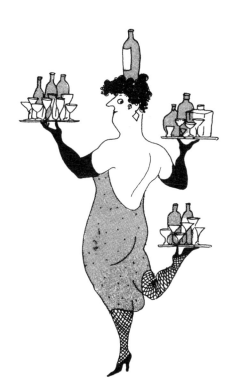

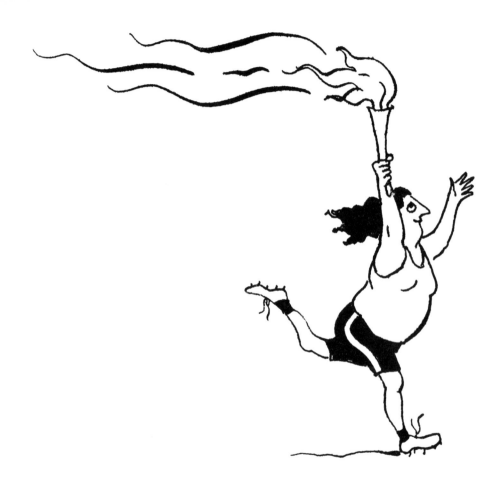

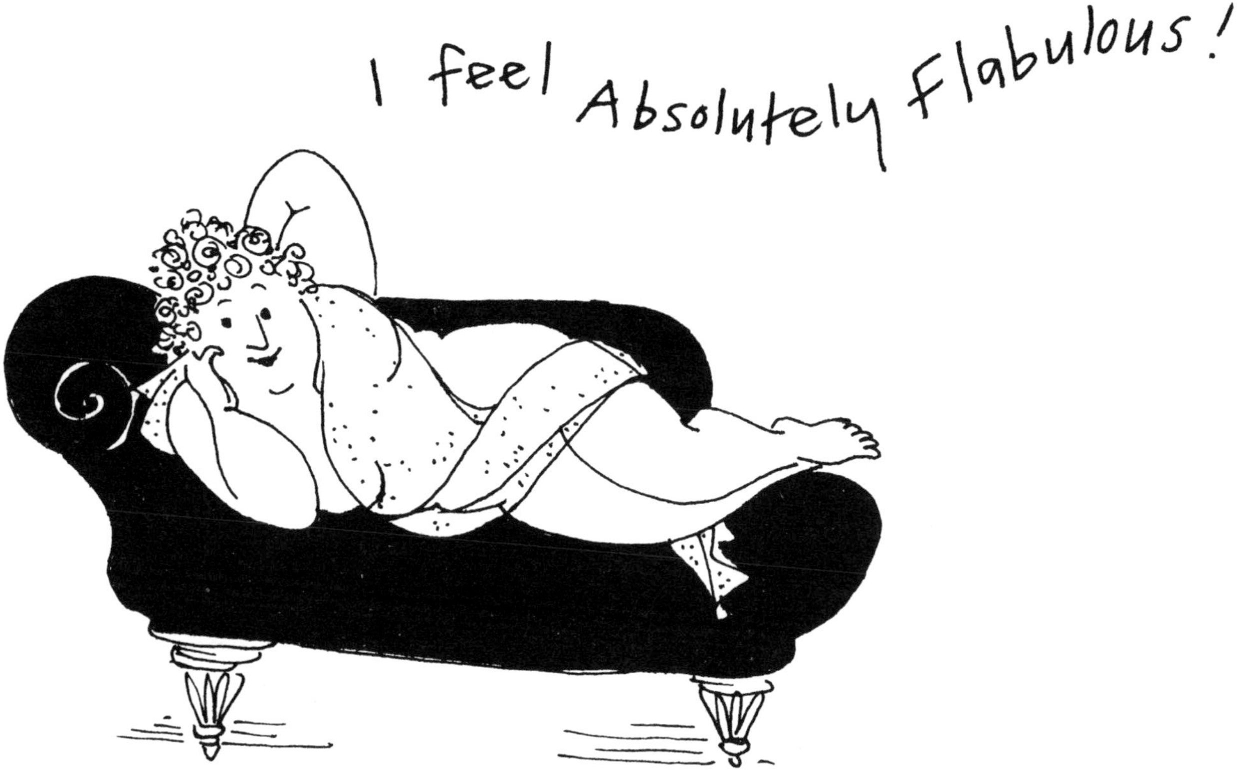
I feel Absolutely Flabulous!

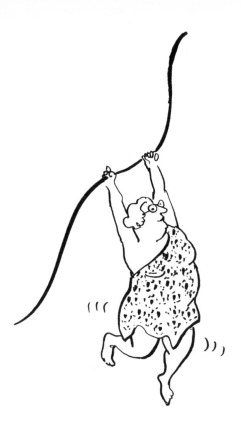

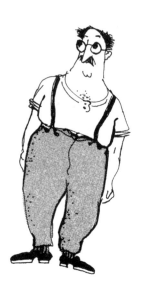

DANGER
SIGNALS

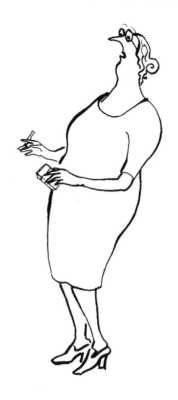

it's time to worry when...

... you develop strange symptoms ....

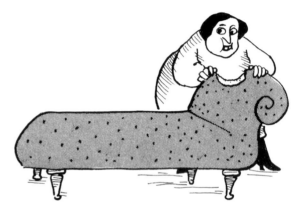

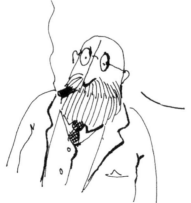

An unusual eating disorder, you say ? Could you be more specific ?

... invitations bring on hysteria...

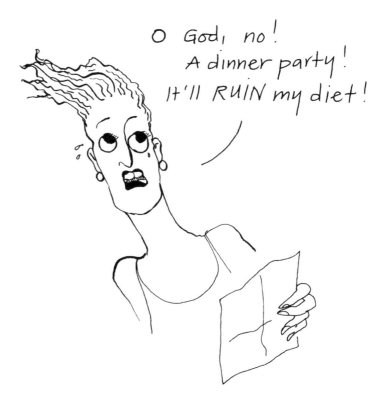

O God, no!
A dinner party!
It'll RUIN my diet!

...your friends can't understand you...

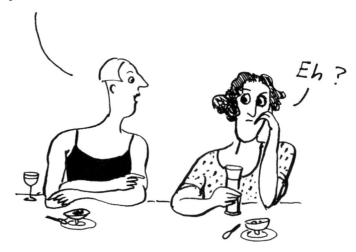

So I usually choose watermelon
for its cancer-beating lycopene,
or strawberries for their
immunity-boosting bioflavanoids...

Eh?

...*you read diet books like novels*...

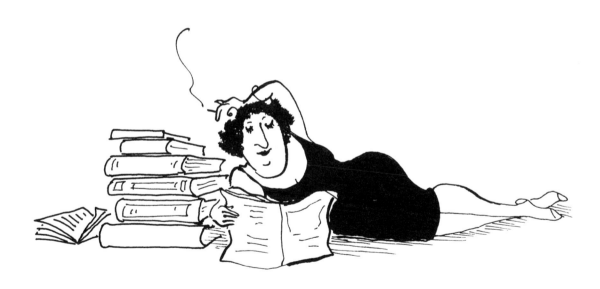

USEFUL TIPS AND GADGETS

Plenty of water
and regular mud-packs,
that's my
secret...

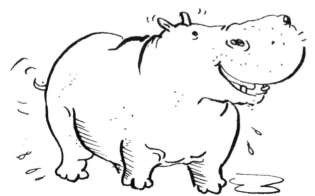

SUCH AS-

... the elastic tape measure ...

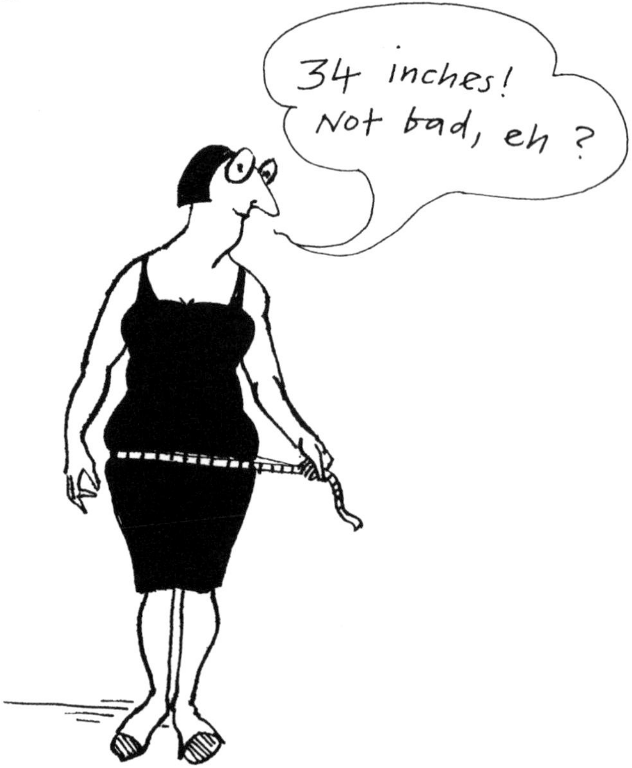
34 inches!
Not bad, eh ?

... scales that (tactfully) speak your weight ...

twelve and a half stone – I've seen worse ...

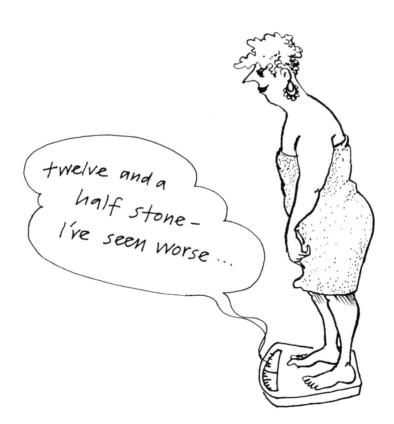

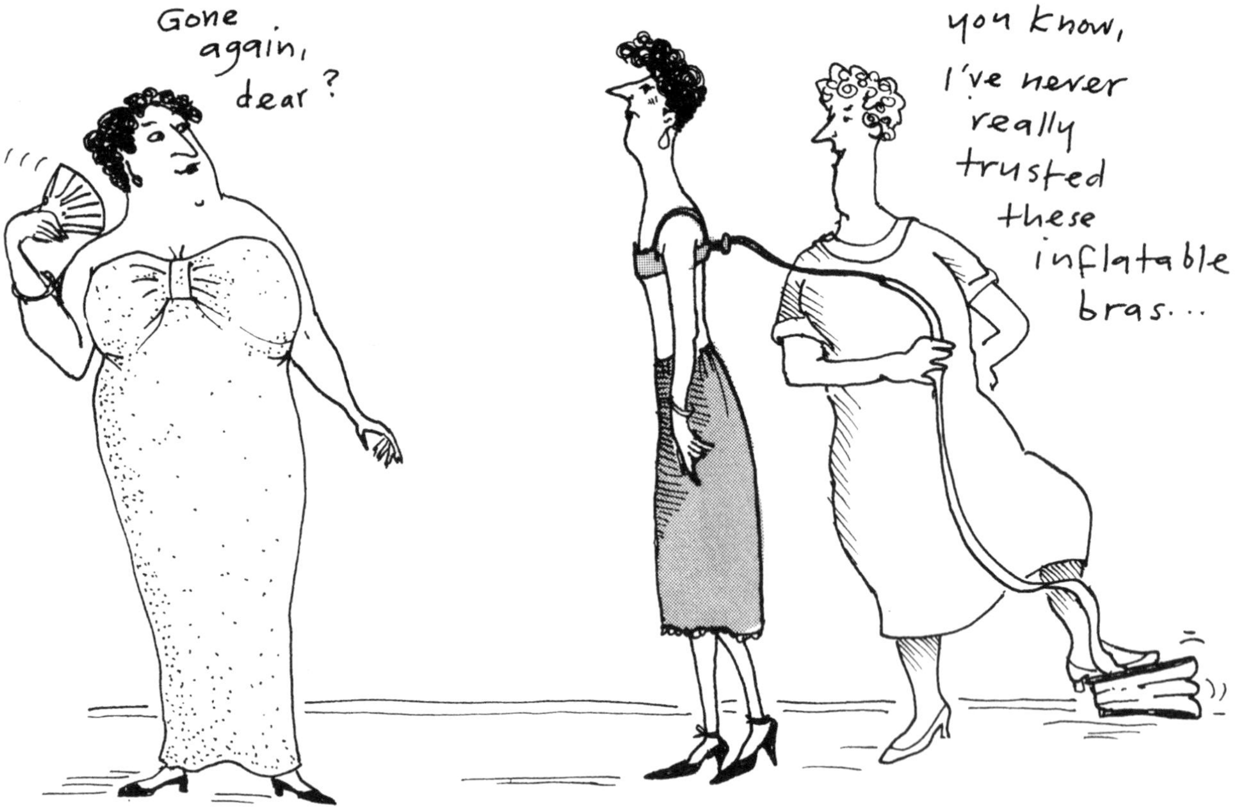
Gone again, dear?
You know, I've never really trusted these inflatable bras...

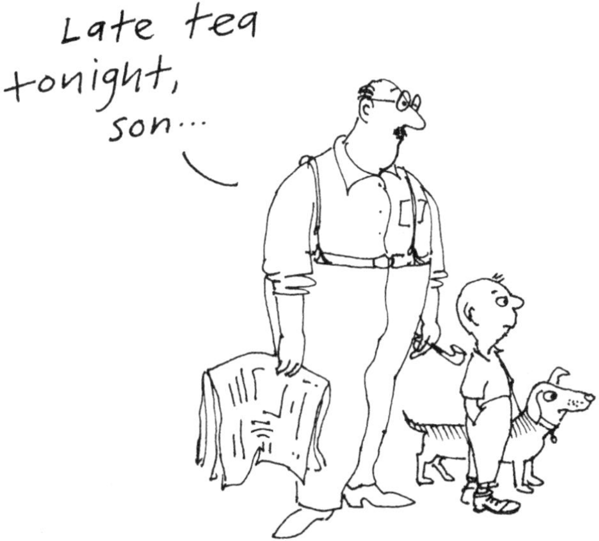

Late tea
tonight,
son...

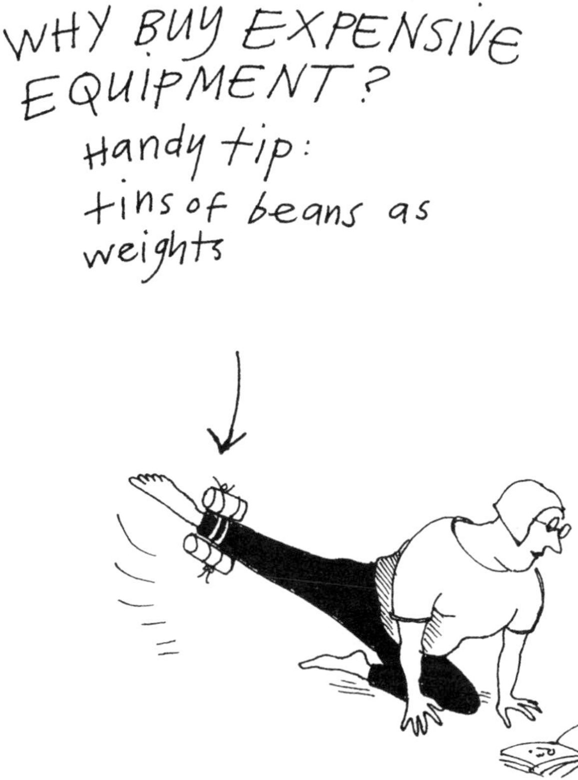

WHY BUY EXPENSIVE
EQUIPMENT?
Handy tip:
tins of beans as
weights

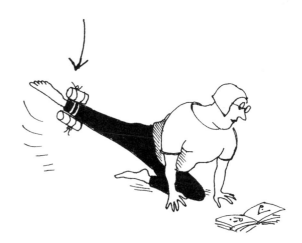

Aerobic food preparation: 1:

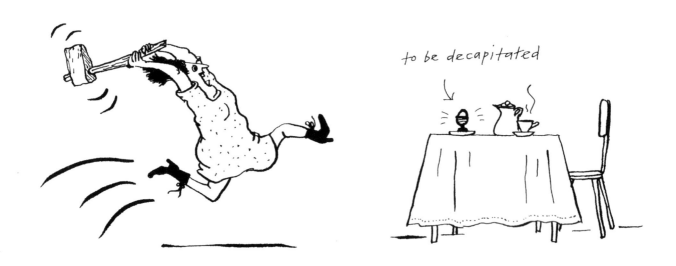

to be decapitated

use up your calories in advance by expending plenty of energy…

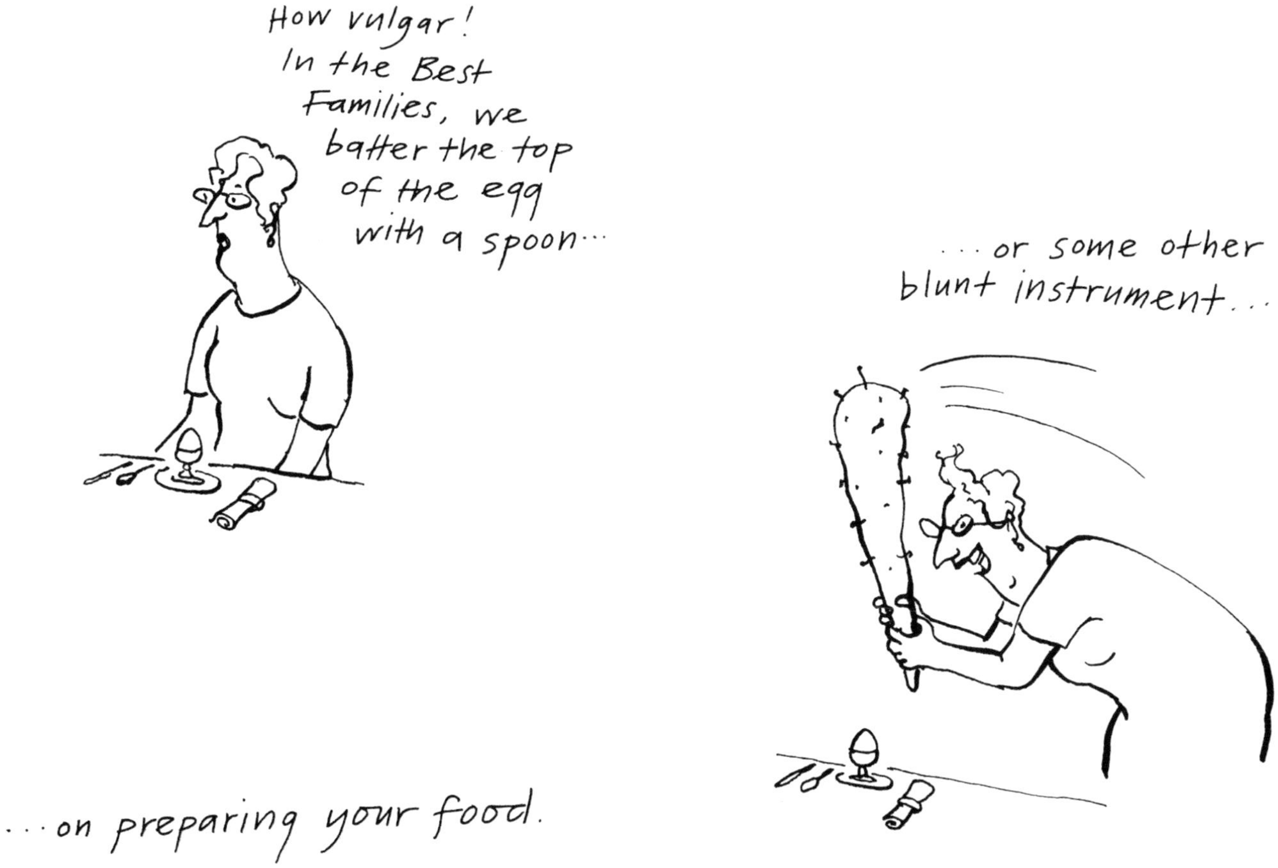
How vulgar! In the Best Families, we batter the top of the egg with a spoon...
...or some other blunt instrument...
...on preparing your food.

Aerobic food preparation: 2:

Fancy a glass of grape juice ?

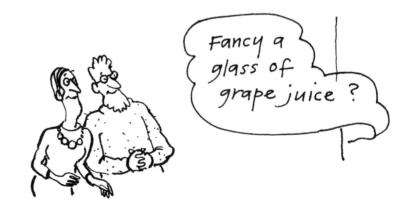

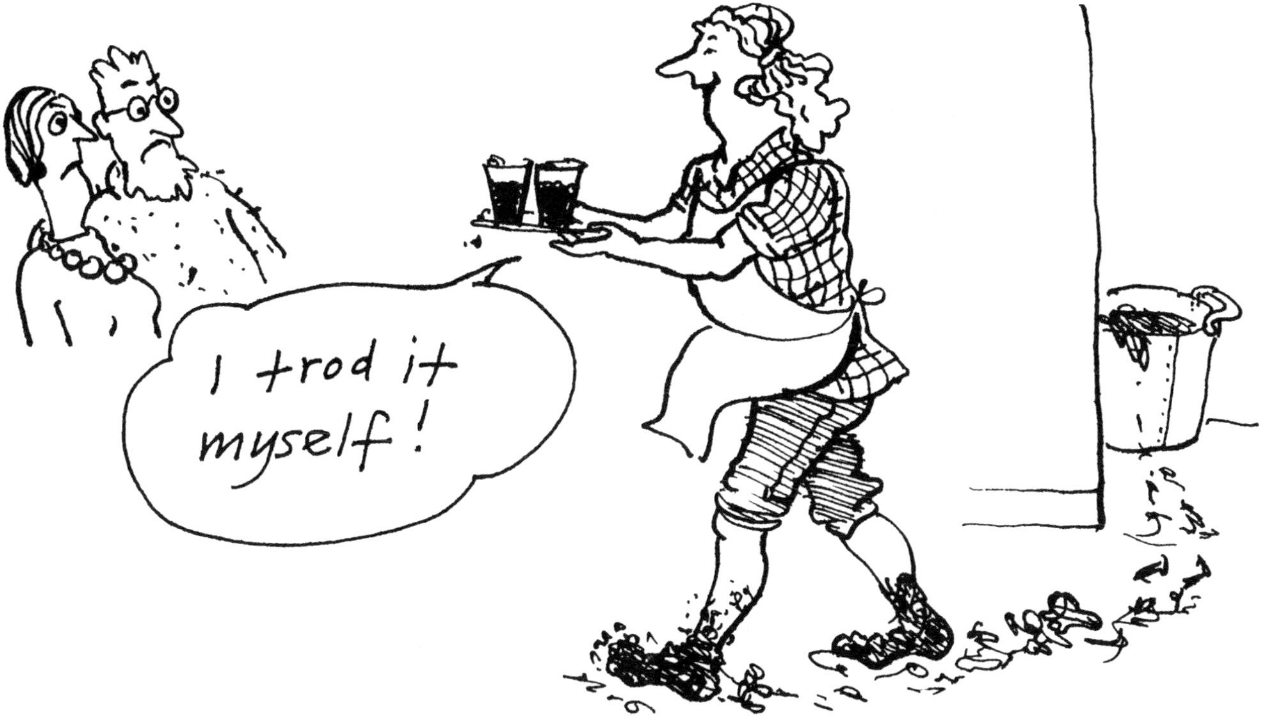
I trod it myself!

Aerobic food preparation: 3:

Come in! I've just knocked up a batch of scones!

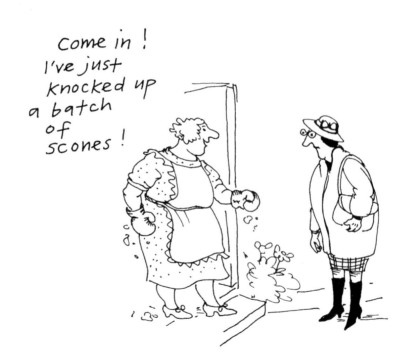

For the successful slimmer:
what to do with those extra-roomy garments...

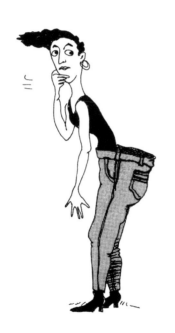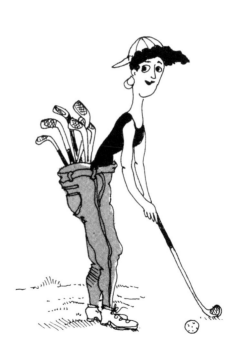

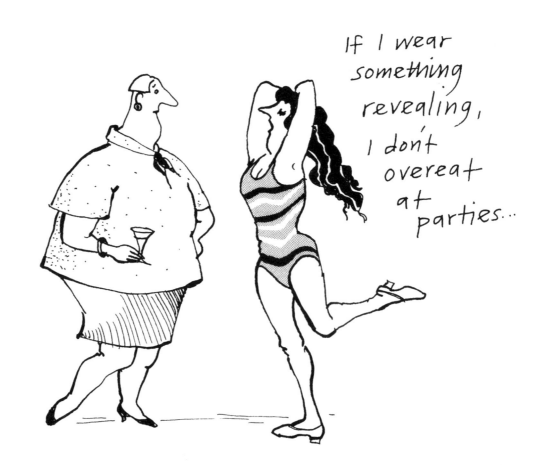

If I wear
something
revealing,
I don't
overeat
at
parties...

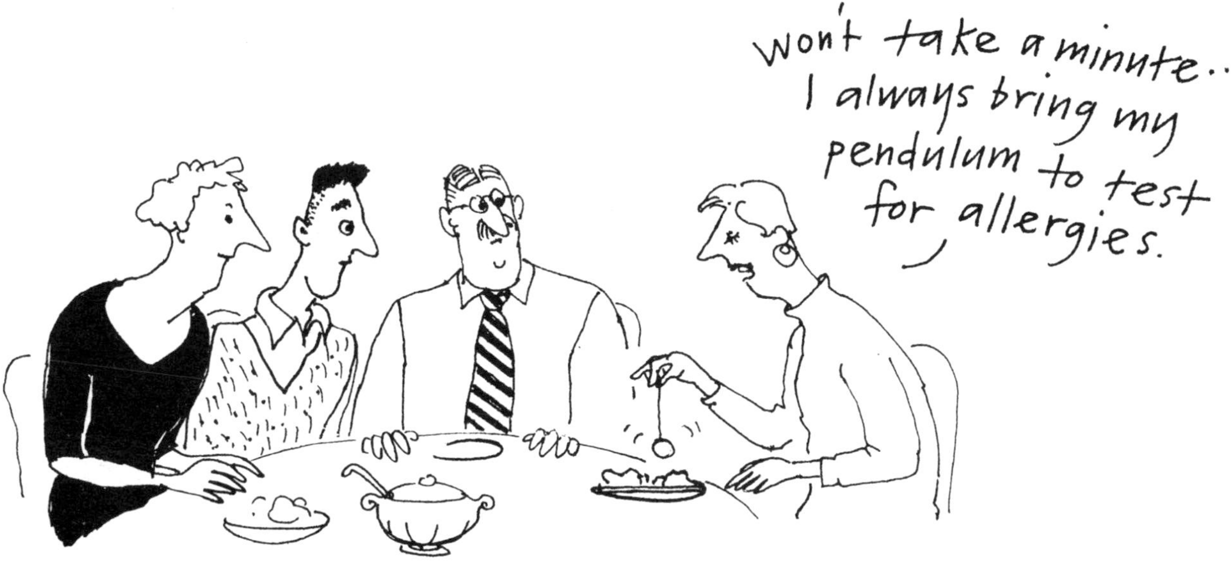
won't take a minute...
I always bring my
pendulum to test
for allergies.

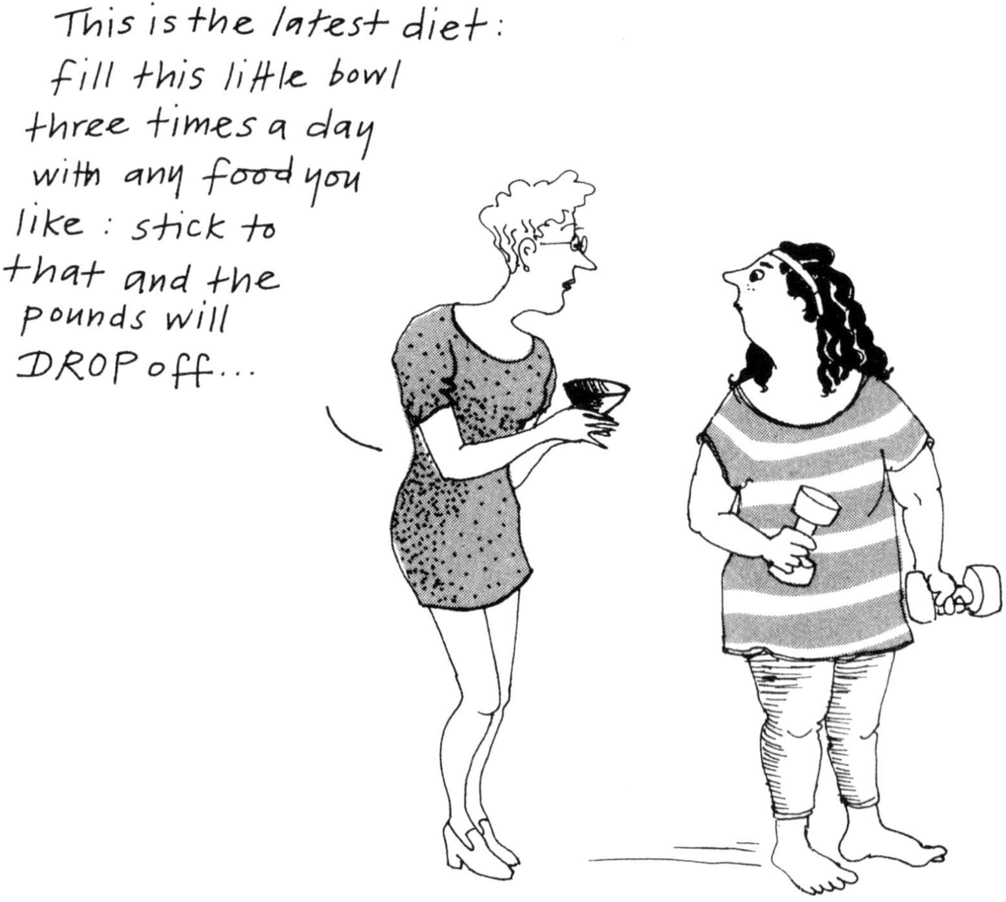
This is the latest diet: fill this little bowl three times a day with any food you like: stick to that and the pounds will DROP off...

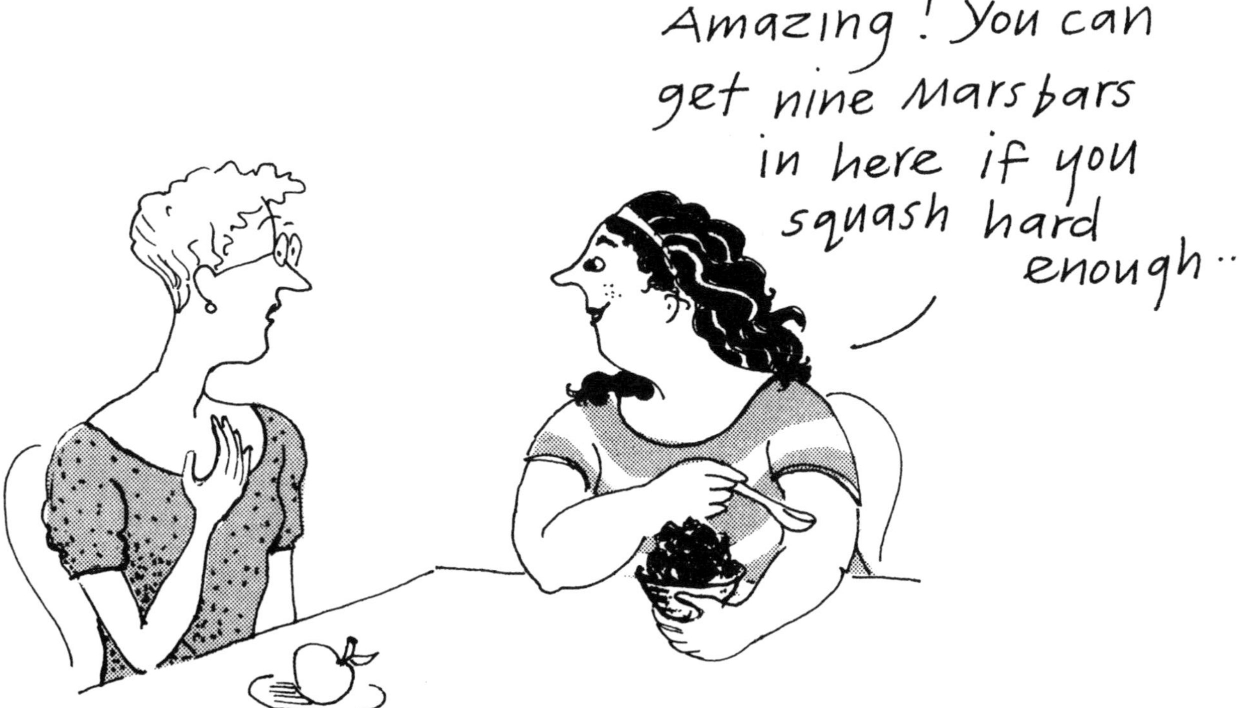
Amazing! You can get nine Mars bars in here if you squash hard enough...

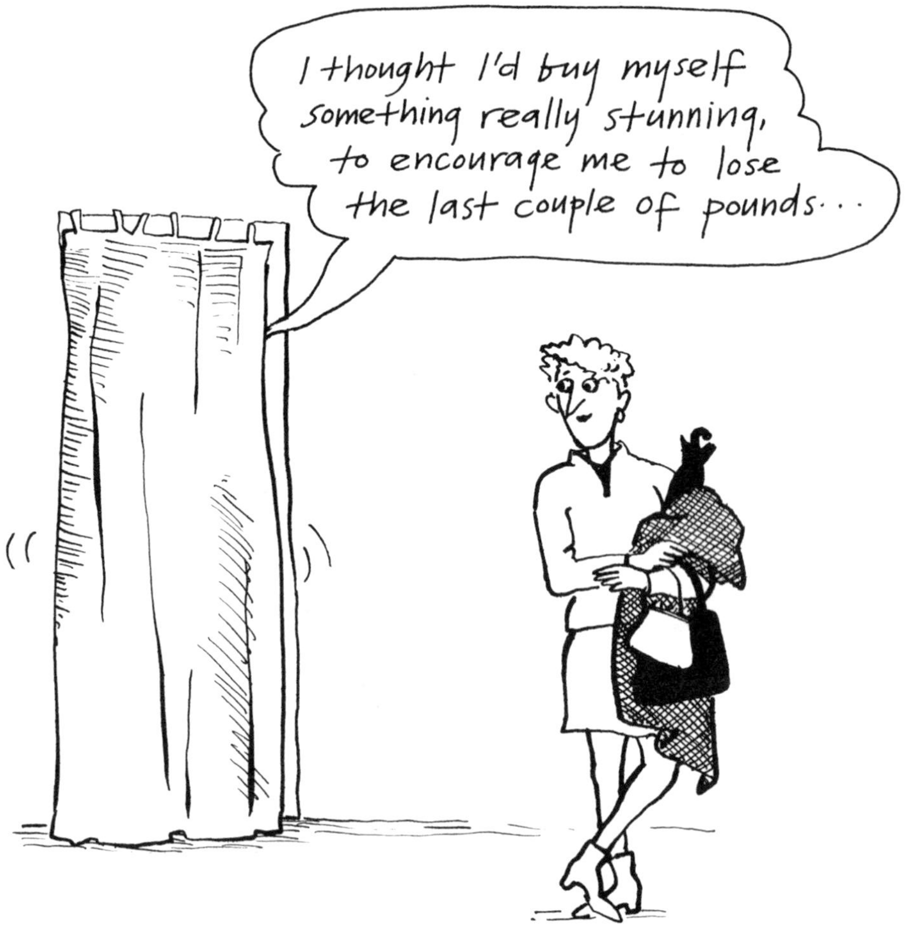
I thought I'd buy myself something really stunning, to encourage me to lose the last couple of pounds...

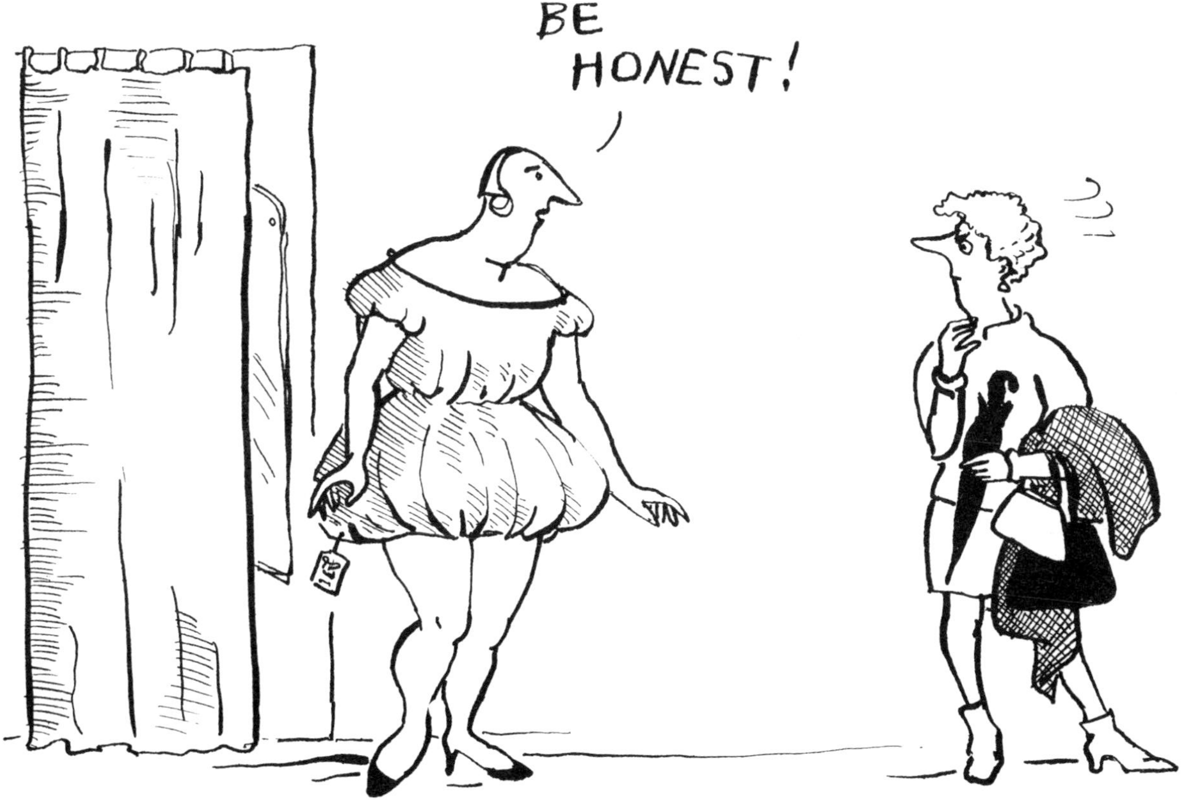
BE HONEST!

THE SOCIAL ROUND

Hop it, Frank - this is Girl Talk !
DIET

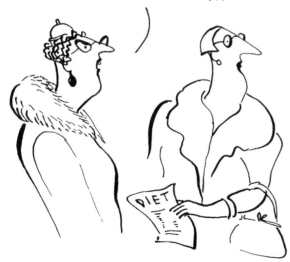

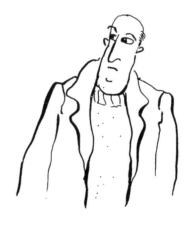

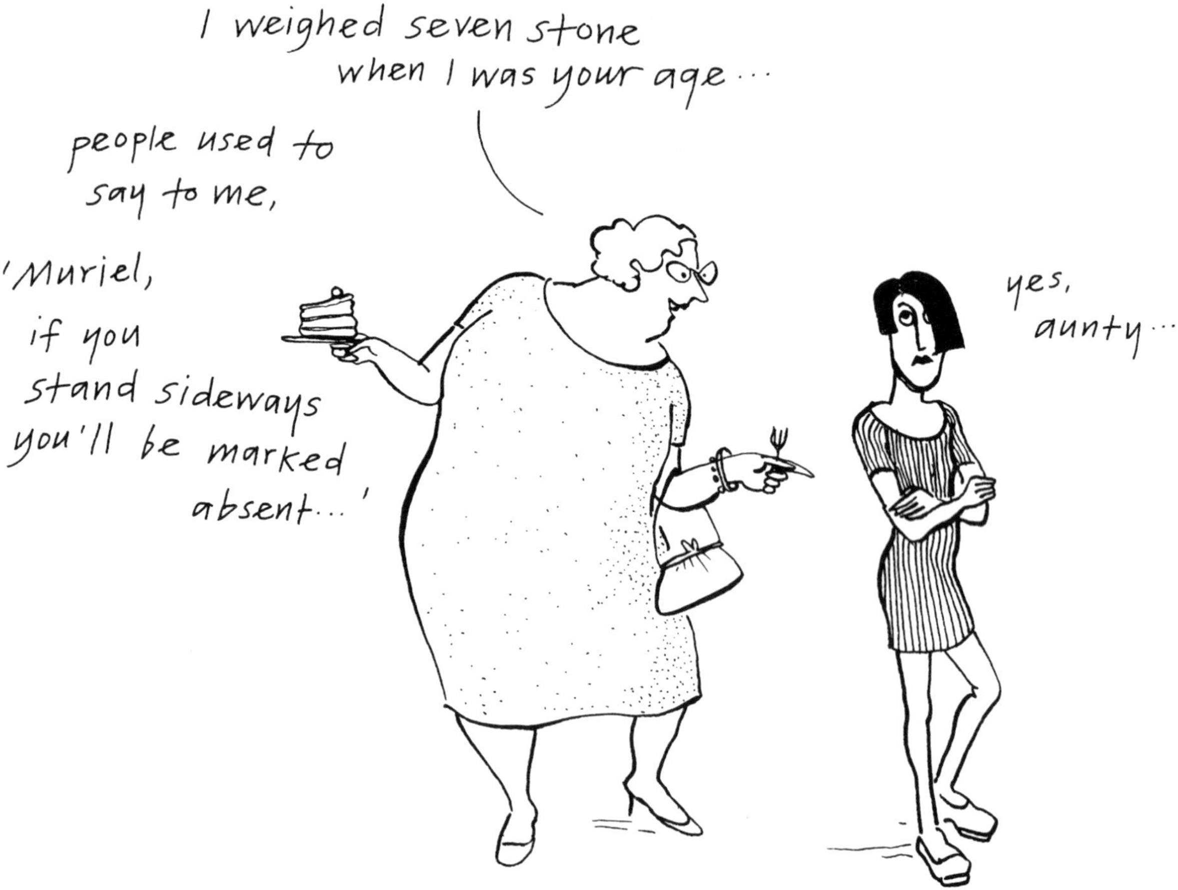
I weighed seven stone when I was your age...
people used to say to me,
'Muriel, if you stand sideways you'll be marked absent...'
yes, aunty...

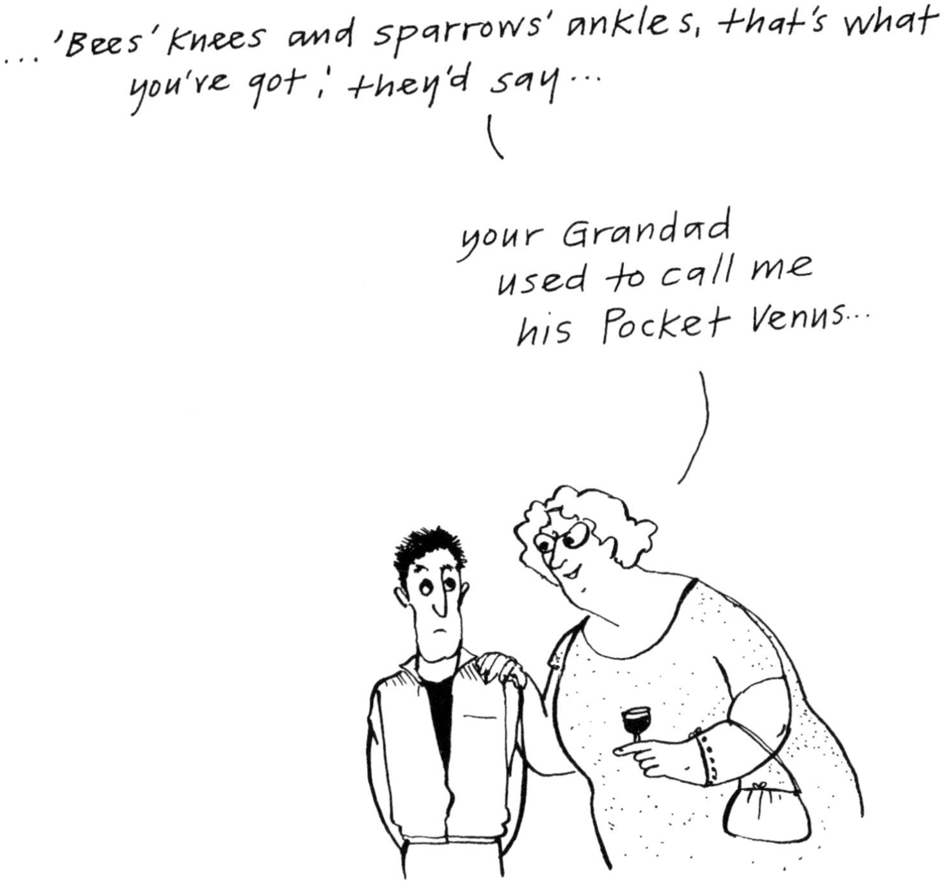
...'Bees' knees and sparrows' ankles, that's what you've got,' they'd say...
your Grandad used to call me his Pocket Venus...

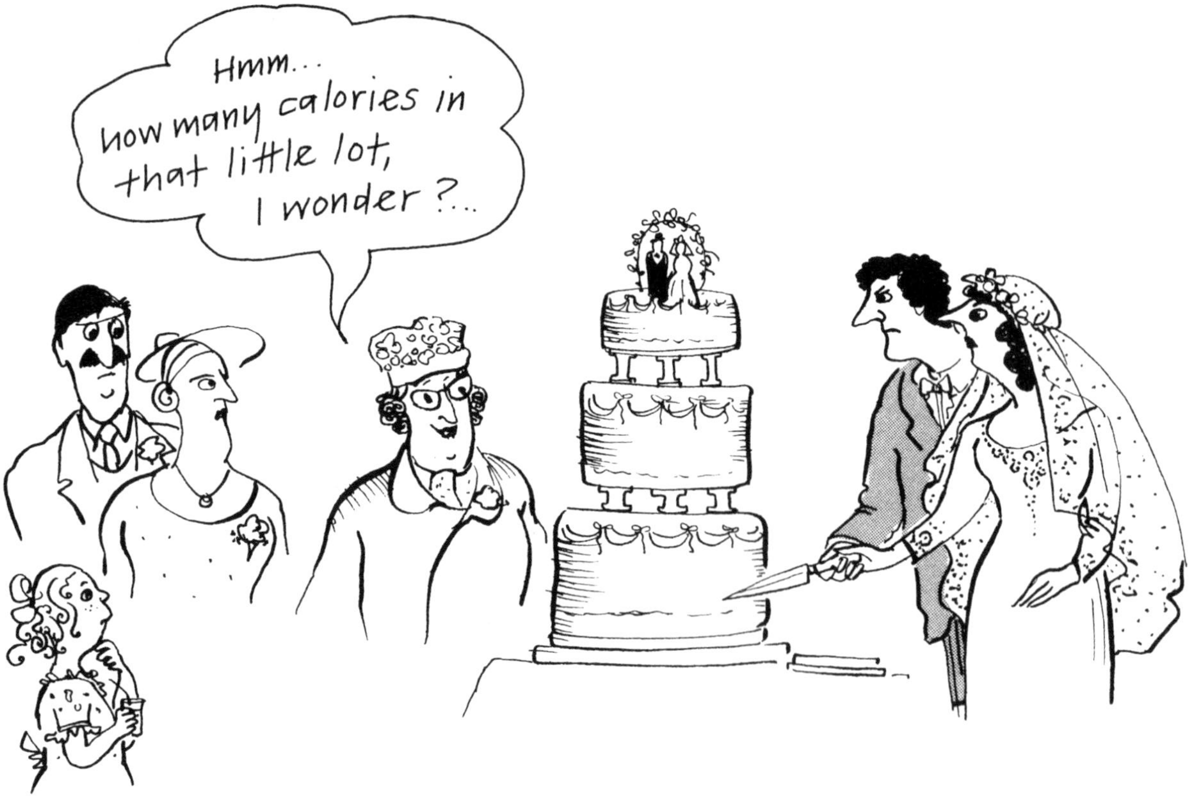
Hmm...
how many calories in
that little lot,
I wonder ?...

SPOILSPORT: 1

Hmm... could do with a bit of work on her lower abdominals...

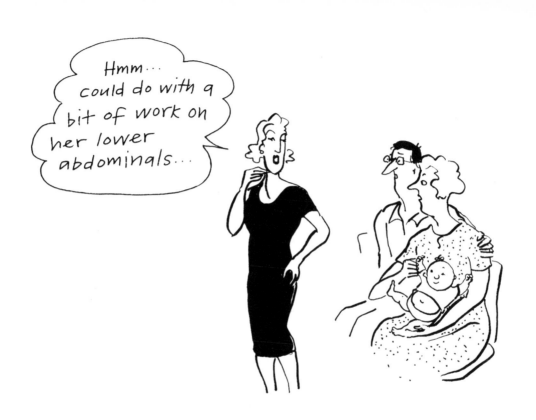

SPOILSPORT : 2

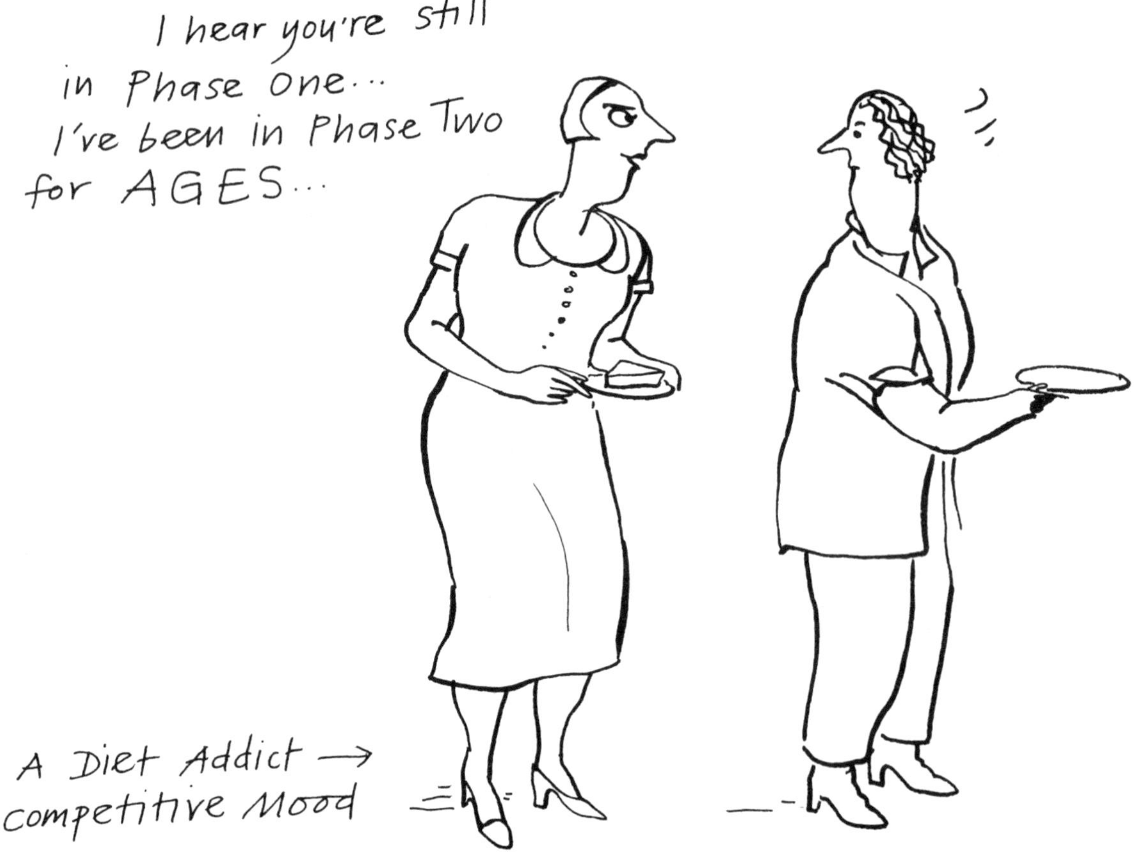
I hear you're still
in Phase One...
I've been in Phase Two
for AGES...
A Diet Addict →
in competitive Mood

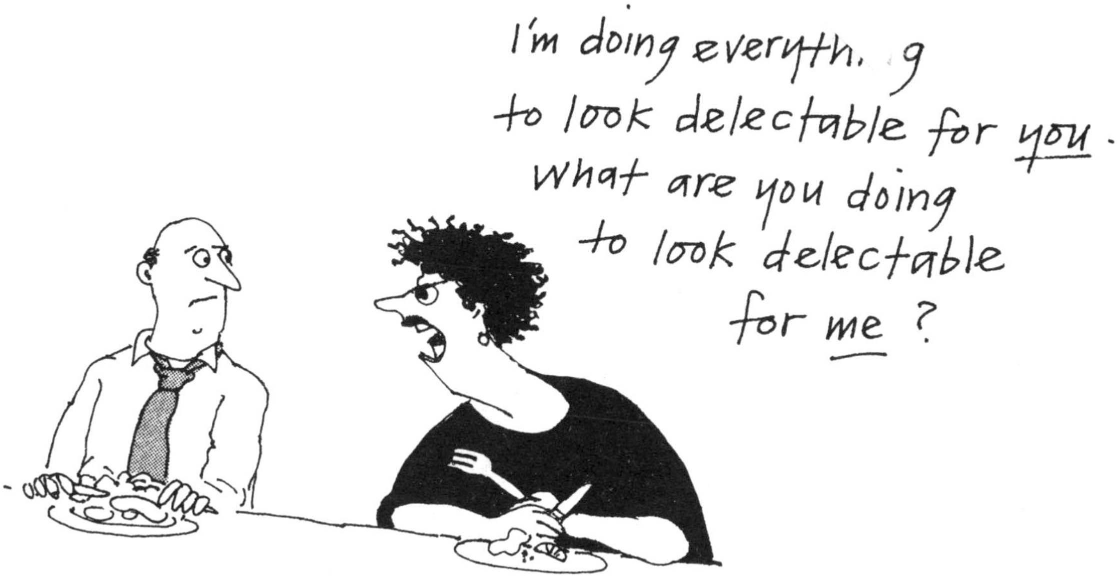
I'm doing everything
to look delectable for you.
What are you doing
to look delectable
for me?

Another Diet Addict in Competitive Mood

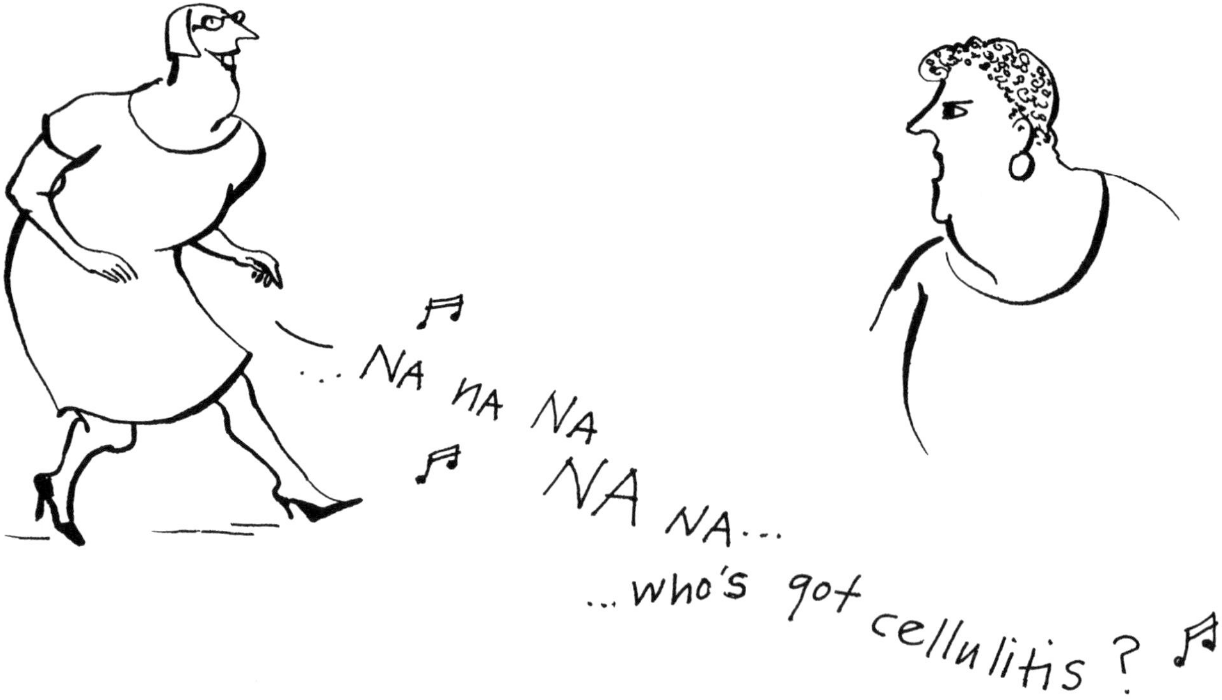
...NA NA NA
NA NA...
...who's got cellulitis?

yet another DIet Addict in Competitive Mood

FAT?
I prefer to call it
AVOIRDUPOIS !

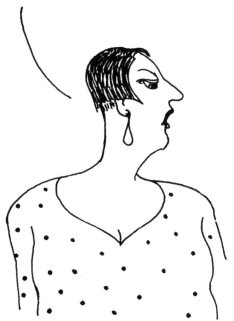

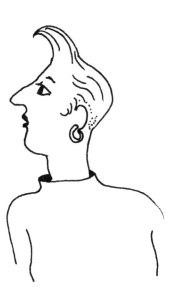

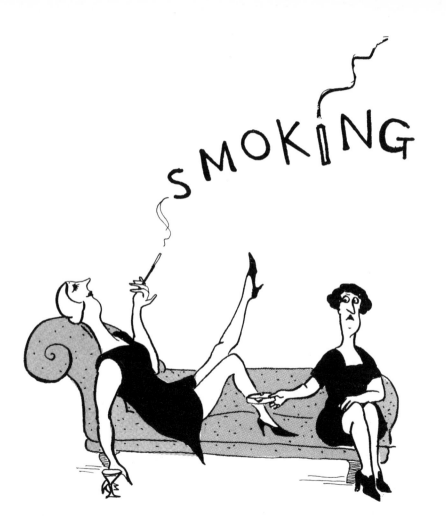

SMOKING

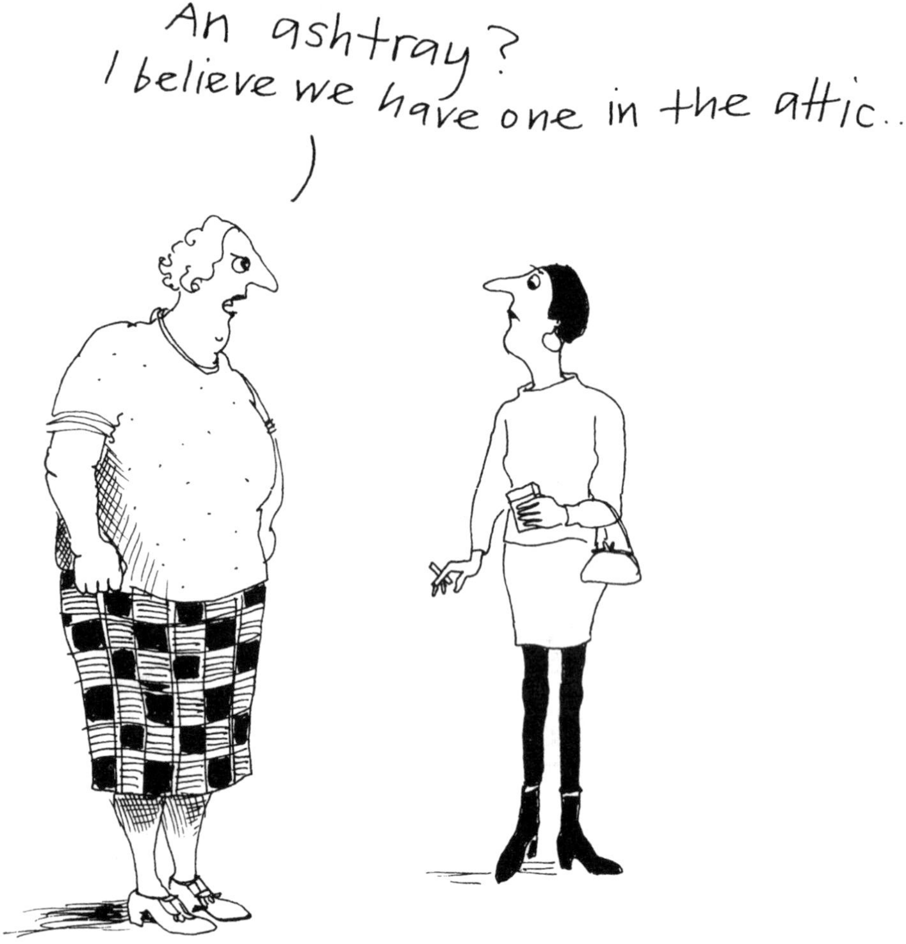
An ashtray?
I believe we have one in the attic...

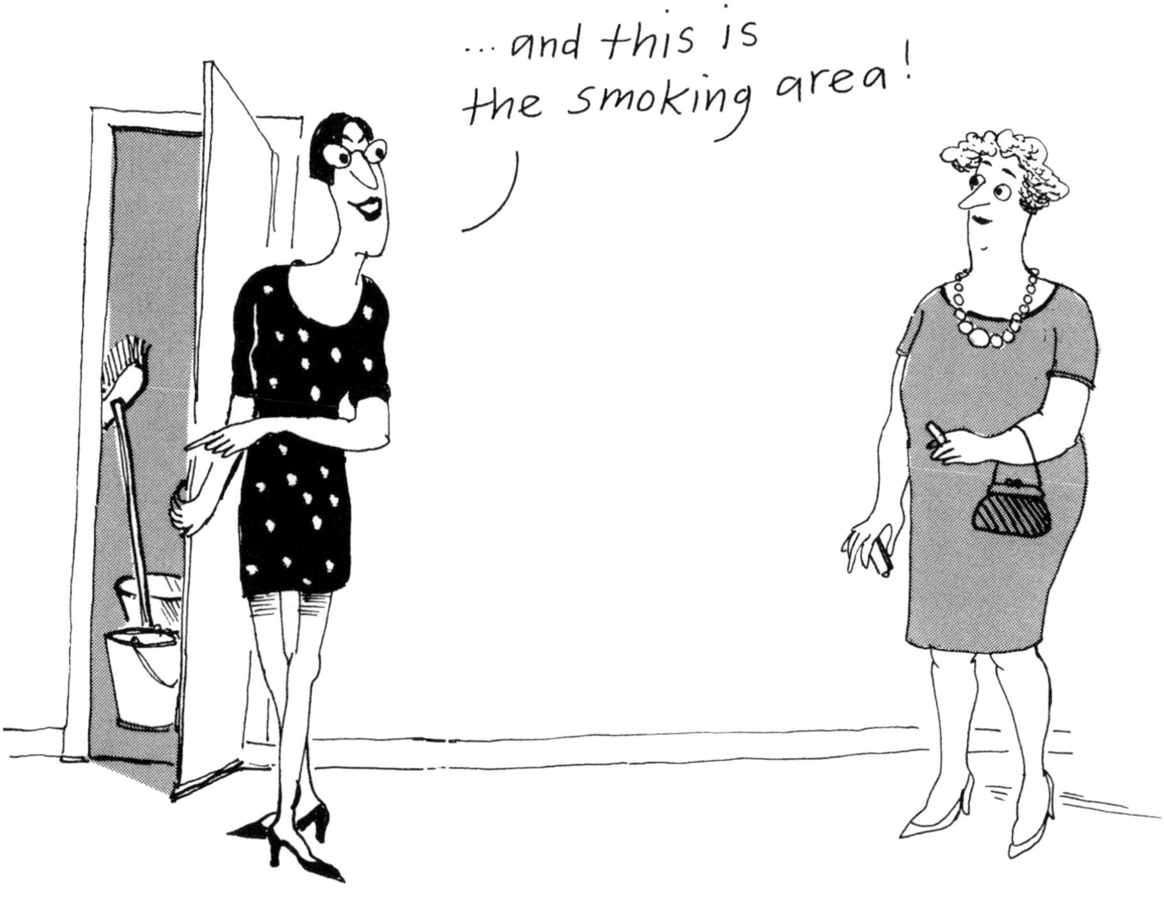
...and this is the smoking area!

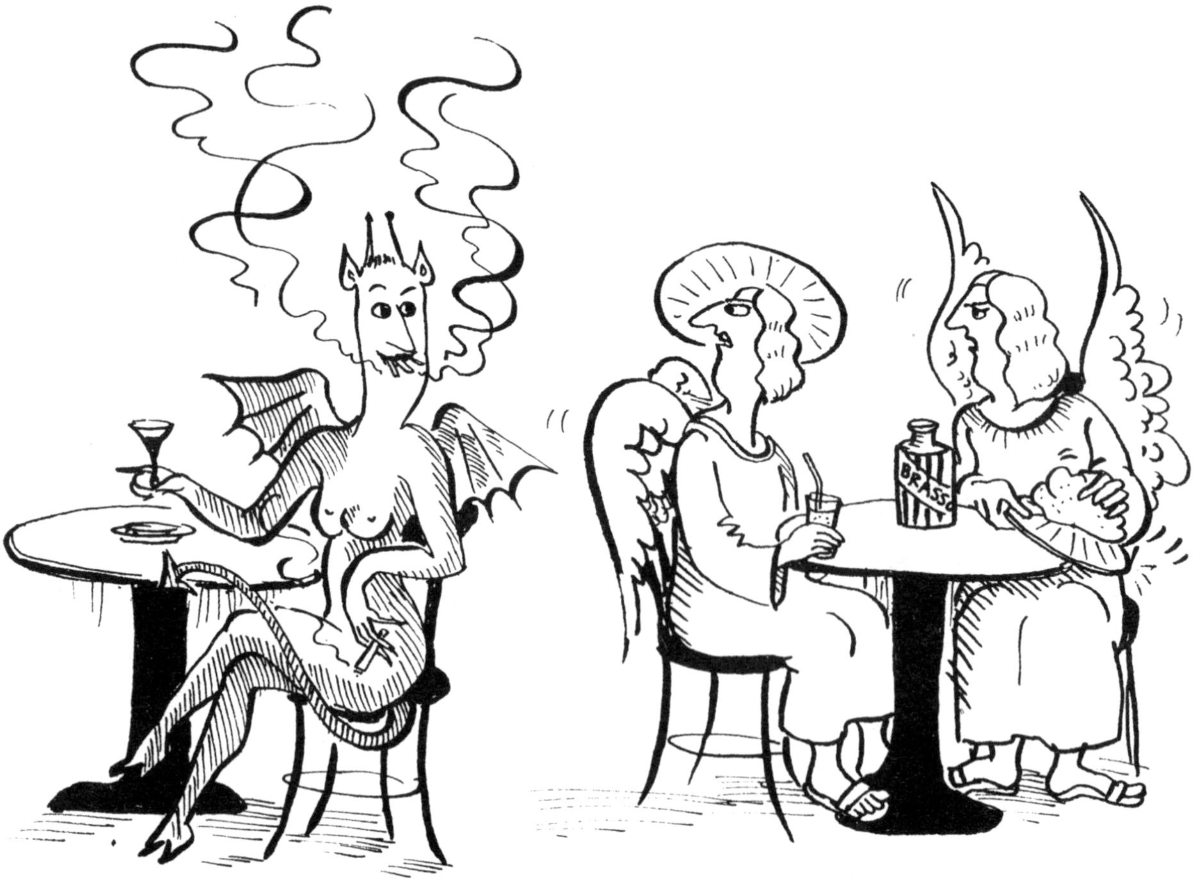
BRASSO